THERAPEUTICS IN TERMIN

THERAPEUTICS IN TERMINAL CANCER

Robert G Twycross MA, DM, FRCP
Macmillan Clinical Reader in Palliative Medicine, University of Oxford
Consultant Physician, Sir Michael Sobell House, Churchill Hospital, Oxford
Director, WHO Collaborating Centre for Palliative Cancer Care, Oxford, UK

Sylvia A Lack MB, BS
Director, Chronic Pain Syndrome Rehabilitation Program and Attending
Physician, Spinal Cord Unit, Gaylord Hospital, Wallingford, Connecticut
Consultant in Hospice Care, St. Mary's Hospital, Waterbury, Connecticut
Attending Physician, World War II Memorial Hospital, Meriden, Connecticut, USA

SECOND EDITION

CHURCHILL LIVINGSTONE
EDINBURGH LONDON MELBOURNE AND NEW YORK 1990

CHURCHILL LIVINGSTONE
Medical Division of Longman Group UK Limited

Distributed in the United States of America by
Churchill Livingstone Inc., 1560 Broadway, New York,
N.Y. 10036, and by associated companies, branches and
representatives throughout the world.

First published 1984 (Pitman Publishing Ltd)
   Reprinted 1986 (Churchill Livingstone)
   Reprinted 1987
   Reprinted 1988
Second edition 1990
   Reprinted 1990

ISBN 0-443-04118-0

British Library Cataloguing in Publication Data
Twycross, Robert G. (Robert Geoffrey)
   Therapeutics in terminal cancer.–2nd ed.
   1. Man. Terminal cancer. Symptoms. Drug therapy
   I. Title II. Lack, Sylvia A.
   616.99'4047

Library of Congress Cataloging in Publication Data
Twycross, Robert G.
   Therapeutics in terminal cancer/Robert G. Twycross.
Sylvia A. Lack.–2nd ed.
   Includes index.
   1. Cancer–Palliative treatment. 2. Cancer–Complications and
sequelae–Treatment. 3. Cancer pain–Treatment. 4. Terminal care
I. Lack, Sylvia A.´II. Title
   [DNLM: 1. Neoplasms–therapy–handbooks. 2. Palliative
Treatment–handbooks. 3. Terminal Care–handbooks. OZ 39 T975t]
RC271.P33T89 1990'
   616.99'406–dc20

Produced by Longman Singapore Publishers (Pte) Ltd
Printed in Singapore

FOREWORD

'I knew I needed attention' is the revealing phrase in which many patients in the terminal stages of cancer have summed up their needs. Although symptom control is increasingly recognized as a respectable branch of therapeutics, there are still too many terminally ill patients who receive the message that nothing more can be done. Failure to analyse a patient's physical distress, or its inept treatment, also means that other elements of his total suffering, emotional, social or spiritual, are not recognized or alleviated. In consequence, he never achieves the potential that may still remain to him. This book, coming from two writers of wide experience in both general internal medicine and terminal care, shows how meticulous attention to detail can lead to appropriate and effective treatment to the end of a patient's life. This transforms his experience, and the memories of his family.

The authors offer 'a framework of knowledge from which a doctor can develop an individual therapeutic approach'. Coming from two special centres and general hospitals on both sides of the Atlantic it distils knowledge culled from a sustained search for quality of care to give quality of life even in the midst of dying. It will stimulate the reader to look and look again at what he can add to its many suggestions as he develops his own practice in this demanding and rewarding field.

Particularly helpful is the well-researched section, 'Oral morphine in advanced cancer'. This should effectively dispel many of the myths that continue to deny relief to patients with terminal pain. May we perhaps also hope that it will encourage a greater readiness to consider the use of narcotics in other fields. The often puzzling area of neuropsychological symptoms is well opened up by the authors' painstaking methods; for example, confusion and dementia are clearly distinguished and a variety of suggestions made to help clarify the treatment of states that can be so distressing to families. An introduction to some of the psychosocial issues was to be expected from two doctors who have consistently appreciated their importance and is interesting reading in their orderly note form. The importance of team work, the doctor's commitment to the family as well as to his patient and the whole place of a terminal illness as a part of life are shown in their place alongside the challenge to therapeutic skill.

Those of us who have participated in any way in the development of this branch of medicine will recognize this book as an important contribution, summing up with rare economy the present state of knowledge and encouraging its readers to continue to develop their own skills. It is a fascinating example of a reductionism that clarifies confusing situations but returns continually to see the whole, the individual person. The attention needed from the staff caring for each dying person with his own mix of culture, past, personality and relationships will be made far easier for those who use its methods as their starting point.

Cicely Saunders

PREFACE TO SECOND EDITION

In this second edition of *Therapeutics* we have tried to avoid change simply for the sake of change. Even so, apart from the final section on psychosocial issues, much of the book has undergone considerable alteration. Moreover, because about 100 new patients with lymphoedema are seen each year at Sobell House, a new section on this symptom has been introduced. In the section on pain relief, the important division of cancer pain into opioid responsive, semi-responsive and resistant is now clearly enunciated, and more advice about deafferentation pain included. Notice has been taken of the classification of opioids on the basis of receptor affinity and activity. Similarly, the impact of slow-release morphine tablets on prescribing practice has been recognized.

Even though we no longer run the 5-day course referred to in the preface of the first edition, we continue to teach extensively. We still consider *Therapeutics* essentially as lecture notes. For detailed discussion of many of the topics, the reader is referred to our books on *Pain Relief* and *Alimentary Symptoms*.

Acknowledgements

In addition to the stimulus provided by our colleagues, we wish to acknowledge more specifically the help received from a number of people. The recommendations about local anaesthetic congeners and deafferentation pain are largely those of Robert Dunlop. The advice about the care of syringe drivers stems from an educational videotape available from St. Christopher's Hospice. The comments on sympathetic maintained pain owe much to Mark Churcher. Caroline Badger helped considerably in the preparation of the section on lymphoedema. The list of questions in the section on spiritual care comes from Rev. Toshiyuki Kubotera of Yodogawa Christian Hospital, Japan. We are grateful to the Medical Information Departments of a number of pharmaceutical companies for providing data, references and reprints. Finally, we should like to express our gratitude to Kristen Cowcher for reading the text and making many helpful suggestions, and to Karen Jones for repeatedly word-processing the whole of this second edition.

Oxford, 1990

RGT
SAL

PREFACE TO THE FIRST EDITION

The book is essentially a set of seminar and lecture notes, and derives from the joint teaching programme run by the authors. Each year a 5-day residential course of some 60 physicians is held on 'Symptom Control in Far-Advanced Cancer'. The venue alternates between Oxford, England and New Haven, Connecticut. The contents have been updated and expanded to include differences in practice between Britain and America. The original lecture notes on the use of oral morphine have been replaced by a more detailed section, 'Oral morphine in advanced cancer'.

This book is written primarily for doctors. It will, however, be of interest and value to many nurses, particularly those associated with departments of radiotherapy and oncology, or with a hospice. It is possible, too, that clinician-teachers may find the book of value in relation to their own teaching programmes.

The book provides a framework of knowledge from which a doctor can develop an individual therapeutic approach to the control of symptoms associated with far-advanced cancer. The sections headed 'treatment possibilities' contain lists of management strategies for a particular symptom. Physicians must, of course, evaluate the applicability and relevance of each manoeuvre to individual cases using their own professional judgement. Sections headed 'therapeutic plan' or 'recommended drugs' represent the authors' favoured approach.

When using pronouns in reference to patients, the masculine form has been used, in keeping with tradition and simplicity.

Generic names are used to broaden the international usefulness of the book. Only a limited number of proprietary names are included. Readers are directed to publications such as their own National Formulary and, in the USA, the Physicians Desk Reference to ascertain or confirm local Trade options.

The contents of any book cannot be wholly original. We learn much from our pupils, and when sitting at the feet of others. Our appreciation goes to Dame Cicely Saunders for her leadership in this field, and for the personal inspiration she has given to both of us. It was through her that we were drawn into hospice work. Acknowledgement is given to those from other disciplines who have worked together to improve terminal care in the United States of America, notably Shirley Dobihal LPN, Mary Kaye Smith RN, Rev. Edward Dobihal and Dennis Rezendes. We recognize the debt we owe to the many who have helped in the evolution of these pages, especially external members of our course faculty. We thank in particular, in Oxford, Michael Briggs, Geoffrey Hanks, Richard Hillier, Alistair Laing, Averil Stedeford and, in New Haven, David Fischer, Ira Goldenberg, Arthur Knowlton, James Nordlund, Samuel Thier. And, as always, those who have taught us most — our patients and their families.

Oxford, 1984   RGT
                                                                 SAL

ABBREVIATIONS

b.i.d.	twice daily; alternative, b.d.
BP	British Pharmacopoeia
cm	centimetre(s)
cGy	centiGray(s), a measure of irradiation
daily	once a day
dl	decilitre(s) (100 ml)
g	gram(s)
h	hour(s)
Hg	mercury
IM	intramuscular
IV	intravenous
kg	kilogram(s)
L	litre(s)
MAOI	monoamine oxidase inhibitor(s)
mEq	milliequivalent(s)
mg	milligram(s)
ml	millilitre(s)
mm	millimetre(s)
mmol	millimole(s)
min	minute(s)
µg	microgram(s)
NSAID	non-steroidal anti-inflammatory drug(s)
nocte	at bedtime
oz	ounce
PO	*per os*, by mouth
PR	*per rectum*, by rectum
q4h, q6h	every 4 hours, every 6 hours, etc
q.i.d.	four times a day (per 24 hours); alternative, q.d.s.
SC	subcutaneous
SL	sublingual
SR	slow-release
stat	immediately
t.i.d.	three times a day (per 24 hours); alternative, t.d.s.

DRUG NAMES

Generic drug names are generally the same regardless of the country of use. Important exceptions are:

UK	USA
activated dimethicone	simethicone
adrenaline	epinephrine
dextropropoxyphene	propoxyphene
diamorphine (diacetylmorphine)	heroin
frusemide	furosemide
hyoscine	scopolamine
lignocaine	lidocaine
paracetamol	acetaminophen
pethidine	meperidine
urea hydrogen peroxide	carbamide peroxide

In addition readers should note that prednisolone and its inactive pro-drug, prednisone, are identical in potency and efficacy.

All the drugs referred to are not universally available. The reader is advised to check with his own National Formulary or drug compendium if he is in doubt.

* means that a drug or product is available in the UK but not in the USA.

† means that a drug or product is available in the USA but not in the UK.

To Cure *Sometimes*
Relieve *Often*
Comfort *Always*

CONTENTS

CONTENTS

PART ONE

PART ONE

1 SYMPTOM CONTROL

General principles
As death approaches

General Principles

Good symptom control requires clearly defined medical leadership

Attendance by the patient at several different specialist outpatient clinics should be discouraged. Ideally, one team should co-ordinate, direct and explain all aspects of care. Further, both the patient and the family must know to whom they should turn in an emergency.

Patients are often reluctant to bother their doctor about 'minor' symptoms such as dry mouth, altered taste, anorexia, pruritus, cough and insomnia. Enquiries should be made from time to time rather than rely on spontaneous complaint.

Assessment must precede treatment

In cancer patients, the malignant process is not always the cause of a symptom. Moreover, some symptoms are caused by multiple factors. Causal factors include

- Cancer
- Treatment
- Debility
- Concurrent second disorder

Treatment depends on the underlying pathological mechanism

Even when the cancer is responsible, a symptom may be caused in different ways, e.g. vomiting from medication and vomiting from raised intracranial pressure. Treatment may therefore vary from patient to patient.

Explain in simple terms the underlying mechanism(s)

Treatment begins with an explanation by the doctor of the reason(s) for the symptom. This knowledge does much to reduce the psychological impact of the symptom on the sufferer.

- 'The shortness of breath is partly due to the illness itself and partly due to fluid at the base of the right lung. In addition, there is excess fluid throughout the body, particularly in the lungs, and you are slightly anaemic — people with your sort of illness often are. We cannot wave a magic wand and get rid of the underlying tumour — you know that — but this is what we are going to do about the excess fluid...'

If explanation is omitted, the patient may continue to think that his condition is shrouded in mystery. This is frightening because 'Even the doctors don't know what's going on'.

Discuss treatment options with the patient

Whenever possible, the doctor and the patient should decide together on the immediate course of action. Few things are more demeaning to a person's self-esteem than to be disregarded in discussions about him. It is hurtful when staff ignore the patient, treating him as of no importance.

Explain the treatment to the family

Discussion with close relatives usually enlists their cooperation and helps to reinforce symptom control plans. This is vital when the patient is at home. If actively involved in supporting the patient the family have a right to be informed, subject to the patient's approval. It is important, however, not to let the family 'take over'. Whenever possible, the patient's wishes must prevail.

Do not limit treatment to the use of drugs

For example, pruritus is relieved in the majority of patients without resort to antihistamine drugs. Hand cream applied to dry, itching skin several times a day, and soap eliminated in favour of emulsifying ointment is frequently sufficient.

Prescribe drugs prophylactically for persistent symptoms

When treating a persistent symptom with a drug, it should be administered regularly on a prophylactic basis. The use of drugs 'as required' instead of regularly is still the cause of much unrelieved distress.

Keep the treatment as straightforward as possible

When an additional drug is considered, ask the following questions

- What is the treatment goal
- How can it be monitored?
- What is the risk of unwanted effects?
- What is the risk of drug interactions?
- Is it possible to stop any of the current medication?

Seek a colleague's advice in seemingly intractable situations

No one can be an expert in all aspects of patient care. For example, the management of an unusual genito-urinary problem may well be enhanced with advice from a urologist or gynaecologist.

Never say 'I have tried everything' or 'There is nothing more I can do'

It is generally possible to develop a repertoire of alternative measures.

While it is wise not to promise too much, it is important to reassure that you, the doctor, are going to stand by the patient and do all you can.

'No promises but we'll do our best.'

Instead of attempting *immediately* to relieve the symptom completely, be prepared to chip away at the problem a little at a time. When tackled in this way it is surprising how much can be achieved with determination and persistence.

Careful instruction is essential

Precise guidelines are necessary to achieve maximum patient cooperation. 'Take as much as you like, as often as you like' is a recipe for anxiety, poor symptom control and maximum side effects. The drug regimen should be written out in full for the patient and his family to work from (see opposite). Times to be taken, names of drugs, reason for use, (for pain, for bowels, etc) and dose (x ml, y tablets) should all be stated. Also what to do when medication runs out.

Review! Review! Review!

It is often difficult to predict the optimum dose of a symptom relief drug, particularly opioids, laxatives and psychotropic drugs. Moreover, unwanted effects put drug compliance in jeopardy. Arrangements must, therefore, be made for continuing supervision and adjustment of medication.

It is sometimes necessary to compromise on complete relief in order to avoid unacceptable unwanted effects. For example, anticholinergic effects such as dry mouth or visual disturbance may limit dose optimization. Moreover, with inoperable intestinal obstruction, it may be better to aim to reduce the incidence of vomiting to once or twice a day rather than to seek complete control.

Cancer is a progressive disease, and new symptoms occur. It is important that these are dealt with speedily.

Take home medication chart (q4h)

TABLETS/MEDICINES	2 am	On waking	10 am	2 pm	6 pm	Bed-time	PURPOSE

Take home medication chart (q.i.d.)

TABLETS/MEDICINES					PURPOSE

As Death Approaches

With increasing weakness, the patient is faced with the fact that death is inevitable and imminent. Support and companionship are of paramount importance at this time.

Weakness is commonly associated with somnolence or the need to rest for more prolonged periods. Explanation is essential

■ 'This is what often happens in an illness like yours'

[*The doctor understands*]

■ 'When the body is short of energy it takes a lot more effort to do even simple jobs. This means that you will need to rest more in order to restock your limited energy supply'

[*The patient understands*]

For the patient who has not yet come to terms with the situation:

■ 'I think a few quiet days in bed are called for. If tomorrow or the next day you are feeling more energetic, of course you should get up but, for the moment, bed is the best place for you'

[*Not destroying hope, breaking bad news gently, giving the patient permission to let go*]

For the spouse and close family:

■ 'This weakness is quite normal as his body is using all its energy to fight the tumour'

[*The patient is not to blame, he is still fighting. Also he is normal, not peculiar, odd or bad*]

■ 'I think the illness is beginning to win'

[*Time is short*]

Although you may feel powerless in the face of rapidly approaching death, the patient is generally more realistic. He knows you cannot perform a miracle; he appreciates that time is limited.

■ Continue to visit

■ Quietly indicate that: 'At this stage the important thing is to keep you as comfortable as possible'

■ Simplify medication: 'Now that your husband is not so well, he can probably manage without the heart tablets'

■ Arrange for medication to be given sublingually, per rectum or by injection when the patient cannot swallow

■ Continue to inform the family of the changing situation:
  □ 'He is very weak now, but may still have several days'
  □ 'Although he seems better today, he is still very fragile. He could quickly deteriorate and die in a few hours'

■ Control agitation even if it results in sedation

■ Listen to the nurses

2 PAIN RELIEF

Pain and cancer
Treatment modalities
Response to opioids
Use of analgesics
Improving drug compliance
Aspirin
Oral morphine
Continuous SC infusion

Classification of opioids
Buprenorphine
Radiation therapy
Corticosteroids
Deafferentation pain
Sympathetic maintained pain
Pain terms

Pain and Cancer

■ Pain and cancer are not synonymous
  □ ⅔ of patients experience pain
  □ ⅓ of patients do not experience pain

■ Multiple, concurrent pains are common
  □ ⅕ have only one pain
  □ ⅘ have 2 or more pains
  □ ⅓ have 4 or more pains

■ Pain in cancer may be related to:
  □ cancer
  □ cancer treatment
  □ debility
  □ concurrent disorder

Top ten pains in patients with cancer at Sobell House

Nature of pain	Cause
Bone ⎫	
Nerve compression ⎬	Cancer
Soft tissue	
Visceral ⎭	
Myofascial ⎫	Debility
Constipation ⎬	
Muscle spasm	Cancer/debility
Low back pain	Concurrent disorders
Chronic postoperative	Treatment
Capsulitis of shoulder	Debility

Initial Assessment

Because a person has cancer, it does not mean that the
malignant process is the cause of the pain.

Treatment varies according to the cause of the pain; use a
body chart to record sites and probable mechanisms (see
p. 13).

Pain is a somatopsychic experience best defined as 'what the
subject says hurts'.

The perception of pain is modulated by

- The patient's **MOOD**

- The patient's **MORALE**

- The **MEANING** of the pain for the patient

Attention must be paid to factors that modulate pain threshold.

Pain may remain intractable if mental and social factors are
ignored (see p. 14).

Pain is felt more intensely when it lacks positive meaning and
has no foreseeable end. Even when the patient understands
and accepts the diagnosis and prognosis, the course of the
illness means that any pain is seen as a (negative) threat to his
way of life and to his existence. This contrasts with the useful
(positive) warning function of acute pain.

Overprinted body chart

Sites and mechanisms of pain

Present Medication

Other relevant data

How adequate?

Nights

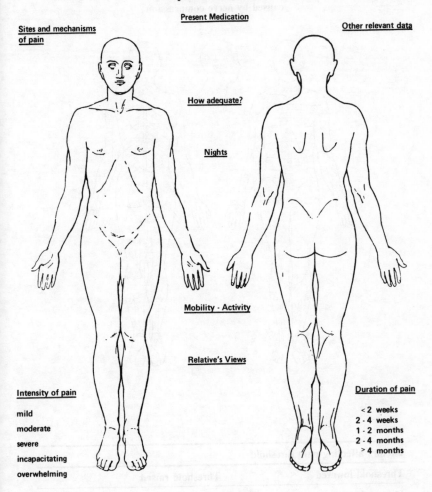

Mobility - Activity

Relative's Views

Intensity of pain

mild

moderate

severe

incapacitating

overwhelming

Duration of pain

< 2 weeks
2 - 4 weeks
1 - 2 months
2 - 4 months
> 4 months

Body chart showing dermatomes. This is necessary when assessing pain caused by nerve compression

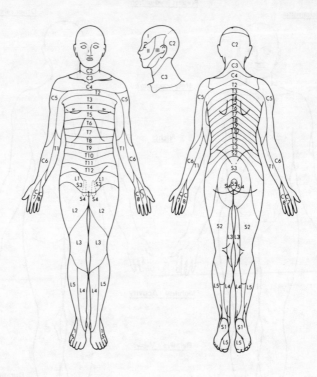

Factors affecting pain threshold

Threshold lowered	Threshold raised
Discomfort	Relief of symptoms
Insomnia	Sleep
Fatigue	Rest
Anxiety	Sympathy
Fear	Understanding
Anger	Companionship
Sadness	Diversional activity
Depression	Reduction in anxiety
Boredom	Elevation of mood
Introversion	
Mental isolation	Analgesics
Social abandonment	Anxiolytics
	Antidepressives

Reassessment

Relief of pain should be assessed in relation to comfort achieved

- During the night
- In the daytime at rest
- On movement

Reassessment remains a continuing necessity; old pains may get worse and new ones may develop.

REVIEW!   REVIEW!   REVIEW!

Common Mistakes in Cancer Pain Management

- Failure to distinguish between pains caused by cancer and pain related to other causes
- Failure to assess each pain individually and to plan separate treatments if necessary
- Failure to use non-drug treatments, particularly for muscle spasm pain
- Lack of awareness that some pains are not relieved at all by opioid analgesics and that others require combined treatment with morphine and a second drug
- *Laissez-faire* approach to drug 'time-table' and patient-family education
- Changing to an alternative analgesic before optimizing the dose and timing of the previous analgesic
- Combining analgesics inappropriately, e.g. two weak opioids or a strong opioid and a weak opioid
- Belief that pentazocine (Fortral*, Talwin†) is more efficacious than codeine and related drugs
- Failure to appreciate that a mixed agonist-antagonist such as pentazocine should not be used in conjunction with codeine and morphine
- Reluctance to prescribe morphine

- Changing from an alternative strong opioid (e.g. buprenorphine, oxycodone†) to a smaller equivalent dose of morphine

- Reducing the interval between administrations instead of increasing the dose

- Using injections when oral medication is possible

- Failure to monitor and control unwanted effects, particularly constipation

- Lack of attention to psychosocial issues

- Failure to listen to the patient

Treatment Modalities

Relief of pain may be achieved by one or more of the following methods

- Explanation
- Modification of the pathological process
- Elevation of pain threshold
- Interruption of pain pathways
- Modification of pattern of living; immobilization

Much can be done to alleviate pain by explaining the mechanisms underlying the pain (this reduces anxiety) and by a continuing concern for the patient (this raises morale).

Modification of the pathological process by means of radiation, chemotherapy or hormone treatment should be considered, even in advanced cancer. In the dying patient it is important to ensure that the burden of treatment is not worse than the disease.

If disease modifying treatment is prescribed, this does not mean that analgesics should be withheld. Best results are often obtained by using two or more treatment modalities concurrently.

The use of analgesics and other drugs is but one way of elevating the pain threshold, thus reducing perception of pain.

The perception of pain requires both consciousness and attention. Pain is worse when it occupies the patient's whole attention. Diversional activity does much more than just 'pass the time'; it diminishes pain. Professional time sitting on the bed and chatting about non-medical issues is not amorphous psychosocial care. It is directly related to pain management; it raises pain threshold by the introduction of understanding and concern.

If the patient is very anxious and/or deeply depressed, it may take 2–4 weeks to achieve optimum results.

'Interruption of pain pathways' refers to chemical neurolysis (nerve blocks) and neurosurgical techniques (e.g. spinothalamic tractotomy). Such procedures are of value in nerve compression pain that is not relieved by the use of an analgesic and a corticosteroid.

Some patients continue to experience pain on movement despite analgesics, other drugs, radiotherapy and nerve blocks. The situation may be improved by suggesting commonsense modifications to the patient's way of life.

Internal fixation or the insertion of a prosthesis should be considered if a pathological fracture of a long-bone occurs, or threatens. These measures obviate the need for prolonged bed rest, and pain is much reduced. The decision to treat surgically depends on the patient's general condition.

Response to Opioids

From a therapeutic point of view, pain in cancer can be divided into three categories:

■ Opioid responsive, i.e. pain that is relieved by opioids

■ Opioid semi-responsive, i.e. pain that is best relieved by the concurrent use of an opioid and a second drug

■ Opioid resistant, i.e. pain that is not relieved by opioids but may be by other drugs

Types of pain in cancer and implications for treatment

Type of pain	Response to opioids	Drug treatment
Nociceptive		
Visceral	+	
Soft tissue	+/−	Non-opioid + opioid
Bone	+/−	
Nerve compression	+/−	Opioid + corticosteroid
Deafferentation (nerve destruction)	−	Tricyclic drug *or* anticonvulsant *or* local anaesthetic congener
Sympathetic maintained	−	
Muscle spasm	−	Muscle relaxant

■ Although NSAID are superior to paracetamol/acetaminophen in rheumatoid arthritis, data is scanty for metastatic bone pain. Circumstantial evidence suggests that both may be equally effective

■ In cancer, mixed nerve compression-deafferentation pains also occur

■ Use of a corticosteroid may convert a mixed pain into a more opioid responsive nerve compression pain

■ Deafferentation pain associated with *degenerative neurological disorders* is occasionally opioid responsive

■ Non-drug treatments are more important for opioid semi-responsive and opioid resistant pains
  □ Radiation therapy for bone pain
  □ Nerve blocks for nerve compression (minority)
  □ Sympathetic blocks for sympathetic maintained pain
  □ Physical therapy for muscle spasm

Use of Analgesics

'By the mouth'

If a patient can swallow, oral administration is the route of choice.

'By the clock'

Round-the-clock pain requires round-the-clock therapy. This means that analgesics should be given regularly and prophylactically. 'As required' medication is irrational and inhumane.

'By the ladder'

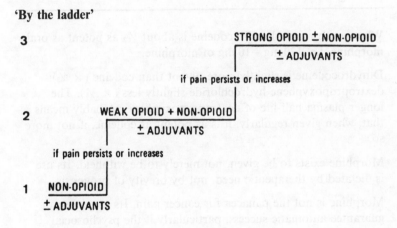

The WHO analgesic ladder for cancer pain management.
(Reproduced by permission of the World Health Organisation)

Non-opioids can be thought of as 'tissue-acting analgesics' and opioids as 'centrally-acting analgesics'. It is good sense to use them in combination, particularly with soft tissue and bone pains.

It is better to use a few drugs well than many badly. The three 'parent' analgesics are aspirin, codeine and morphine. All other analgesics should be regarded as alternatives of fashion or convenience.

If a drug fails to relieve, *move up the ladder*. Do not substitute another drug from the same category.

The 3-step analgesic ladder

Category	Parent drug	Alternatives
Non-opioid	aspirin	paracetamol/acetaminophen flurbiprofen naproxen
Weak opioid	codeine	dextropropoxyphene dihydrocodeine*
Strong opioid	morphine	phenazocine* oxycodone† hydromorphone†

When given regularly q4h, codeine is about $\frac{1}{12}$ as potent as oral morphine, i.e. 120 mg = 10 mg of morphine.

Dihydrocodeine is slightly more potent than codeine ($\times \frac{4}{3}$); dextropropoxyphene hydrochloride slightly less ($\times \frac{7}{8}$). The longer plasma half-life of dextropropoxyphene probably means that, when given regularly, it is as potent as codeine, if not more so.

Morphine exists to be given, not merely to be withheld. Its use is dictated by therapeutic need, not by brevity of prognosis.

Morphine is not the panacea for cancer pain. Its use does not guarantee automatic success, particularly if the psychosocial aspects of pain are ignored.

Do not use pentazocine; it is a weak opioid by mouth and commonly causes psychotomimetic effects.

Pethidine/meperidine (Demerol) and dextromoramide* (Palfium) have little place in cancer pain management because of short durations of action.

Methadone and levorphanol should be used with caution, particularly in the elderly and debilitated. Both may cause drowsiness and confusion when used regularly because of cumulation.

Tolerance to morphine is not a practical problem.

When morphine is used correctly, psychological dependence does not occur.

Physical dependence does not prevent a reduction in the dose of morphine should the pain ameliorate spontaneously or after radiation therapy/nerve block.

Use adjuvant medication

Adjuvant medication is the rule rather than the exception. With opioids, a laxative is almost always necessary and about two-thirds need an antiemetic.

If very anxious, an anxiolytic such as diazepam should be tried; if depressed, an antidepressive.

Improving Drug Compliance

Analgesic regimens should be simple to understand and easy to administer.

It is only necessary to adopt a q4h regimen if a q4h analgesic is prescribed. These include codeine, morphine, diamorphine* and hydromorphone†.

With longer-acting preparations, e.g. flurbiprofen, naproxen, SR morphine sulphate tablets, methadone, buprenorphine, a q4h regimen is *not* indicated. 'After breakfast and at bedtime'; 'on waking, after lunch (and tea), and at bedtime'; 'with meals and at bedtime' will cover all other drug requirements.

If some drugs are best given before meals and others after, pharmacological purity should be foresaken. Opt for one or other time to avoid an impossibly complex schedule. Check drug containers in case the pharmacist has given contrary or complicating advice.

When a q4h dosage regimen is adopted, the first and last doses are linked to the patient's waking time and bedtime. The best additional times during the day are usually 1000 h, 1400 h and 1800 h unless the patient wakes exceptionally late.

The list of drugs and doses for the patient (and family) should be written out clearly (see p. 7). It is useful to add what the different preparations are for, even if this seems obvious to the doctor.

Capsules should be described as capsules and tablets as tablets, not vice versa. Doses should not be described simply as 'spoonfuls'. Patients have been known to use a tablespoon (15 ml) instead of a teaspoon (3.5–5 ml).

A plastic beaker/cup with each 5 ml clearly marked is generally the best way for the patient to self-administer liquid preparations. A calibrated dropper is provided with commercial preparations (e.g. Oramorph*, Roxanol†).

Sometimes, if the above recommendations are carried out, the patient can cope immediately with a new regimen. Not infrequently, however, the patient is found to be in confusion when visited the next day — emphasizing the need for supervision.

Aspirin

Uses

- Analgesic
- Anti-inflammatory
- Antipyretic

Limitations

- Dyspepsia
- Tinnitus
- Deafness

Main Drug Interactions

- Anticoagulant — potentiates
- Oral hypoglycaemic — potentiates
- Corticosteroid — increases gastric irritation
- NSAID — ? antagonizes
- Uricosuric agent — antagonizes

General Comments

- First line analgesic, particularly useful for soft tissue and bone pains

■ Dispersible* (soluble) aspirin causes less gastric irritation/blood loss than standard (non-soluble) tablets

■ Aspirin is more toxic in hypoalbuminaemic patients, as less salicylate is protein-bound

Dosage

■ 600–650 mg is the normal dose. Occasionally 900–1000 mg is used

■ Usually given q.i.d. (with meals and at bedtime) or q4h with morphine. Also 'as required' for intermittent pain

Alternatives to Aspirin

■ If a twice daily preparation preferred, consider the following NSAID:

□ flurbiprofen	100 mg b.i.d.
□ naproxen	500 mg b.i.d.
□ benorylate suspension*	4g/10 ml b.i.d.

■ For patients receiving chemotherapy or with a low platelet count, use a non-acetylated salicylate; these have *no effect* on platelet function and bleeding time:

□ choline magnesium trisalicylate	1000–1500 mg b.i.d.
□ diflunisal	500 mg b.i.d.
□ salsalate	500-1000 mg q.i.d.

Note: Strong NSAID may cause fluid retention, e.g. ankle oedema.

Oral Morphine

■ Morphine sulphate by mouth is the strong opioid of choice for cancer pain

■ Administer in simple aqueous solution (e.g. 10 mg in 10 ml) or as SR tablets

■ If previously receiving a weak opioid, begin with aqueous morphine 10 mg q4h or SR morphine 30 mg q12h

- If changing from alternative strong opioid (e.g. oxycodone†, levorphanol, methadone, buprenorphine) a higher dose of morphine may be needed (see p. 25)

- With aqueous morphine, adjust upwards after first dose if not more effective than previous medication

- Adjust after 24 h if pain not 90% controlled

- ⅔ of patients are pain controlled on 30 mg q4h or less (SR morphine 100 mg q12h). The rest need higher doses, up to 200 mg q4h (SR morphine 600 mg q12h); occasionally more

- With aqueous morphine, a larger bedtime dose (1.5 or 2 × daytime dose) usually enables a patient to go through the night without waking in pain

- Use in combination with a non-opioid for soft tissue and bone pains

- Use in combination with a corticosteroid for nerve compression pains

- Supply an antiemetic for regular use should nausea or vomiting develop, e.g. haloperidol 1.5 mg stat and nocte (see p. 186)

- Prescribe a laxative, e.g. senna and docusate, co-danthrusate* (Normax); casanthranol-docusate† (Peri-Colace). Adjust dose according to response. Suppositories often also necessary

Unless closely monitored, constipation may be more difficult to control than the pain

- Warn patients about possibility of initial drowsiness

- Write out regimen in detail with times to be taken, names of drugs and amount to be taken; arrange for close liaison and follow-up

- If swallowing becomes difficult or vomiting persists, morphine sulphate may be administered by immediate release suppository, or SR tablets may be given PR

- Alternatively, give ⅓ of previously satisfactory dose of morphine as diamorphine hydrochloride* or ½ of previous dose as morphine by SC injection

Approximate oral opioid potency ratios

Drug	Potency ratio	Duration of action (hours)[1]
pethidine/meperidine	1/8	2–3
dipipanone*	1/2	3–5
papaveretum	2/3	3–5
oxycodone†	1	4–6
dextromoramide*	(2)[2]	2–3
methadone	(3-4)[3]	8–12
levorphanol	5	6–8
phenazocine*	5	6–8
hydromorphone†	6	3–4
buprenorphine[4]	60	8

1 Dependent on dose to a certain extent.
2 Dextromoramide — a single 5 mg dose is equivalent to morphine 15 mg (diamorphine* 10 mg) in terms of peak effect but is shorter acting. The overall potency ratio has been adjusted accordingly.
3 Methadone — a single 5 mg dose is equivalent to morphine 7.5 mg (diamorphine* 5 mg). It has a prolonged plasma half-life which leads to cumulation when given repeatedly. This means that when given regularly it is several times more potent.
4 Refers to SL route. In the USA, buprenorphine is available only as an injection.

Continuous SC Infusion

When oral administration is no longer feasible, continuous SC infusion of diamorphine hydrochloride*, morphine sulphate *or* hydromorphone† obviates the need for injections q4h

Indications for Use

- Persistent nausea and vomiting
- Severe dysphagia
- Patient too weak for oral drugs
- Poor alimentary absorption (*rare*)

Advantages

- Constant analgesia — no peaks or troughs.

- Reloaded only once in 24 h

- Comfort and confidence — no repeated injections

- Mobility

- Less nausea and vomiting

Choice of Portable Syringe Driver

- Graseby Medical is a commonly used make in the UK

- Pharmacia is favoured in the USA (more expensive)

- Braun Perfusor — operates by clockwork

If a syringe driver is not available, it may be necessary to insert a butterfly cannula and attach a syringe containing medication for 24 h. The patient, relative, friend or nurse is then instructed to inject 1/6 of the contents q4h. Although this is not a continuous infusion, it does obviate the need for a needle prick several times a day.

Choice of Drugs

Commonly used	Occasionally used[1]	Not suitable
diamorphine*	cyclizine	prochlorperazine[2]
morphine	dexamethasone	diazepam[3]
hydromorphone†	chlorpromazine	
metoclopramide	methotrimeprazine	
haloperidol		
hyoscine		
midazolam		

1 These drugs tend to cause local SC inflammation.
2 Too irritant.
3 Diazepam is oil-based and immiscible with water-soluble drugs.

The frequency with which the needle site has to be changed depends almost entirely on the drugs infused. With an opioid alone ± metoclopramide *or* haloperidol, the injection site may need changing only every 1-3 weeks. If cyclizine or a phenothiazine is added, it may be necessary to change the site daily.

In patients who experience a painful inflammatory reaction the following steps should be considered:

- [ ] change needle site prophylactically, e.g. daily
- [ ] reduce quantity of the irritant drug
- [ ] change to an alternative drug, e.g. cyclizine → hyoscine
- [ ] give irritant drug by IM injection or by rectal suppository q8h
- [ ] place needle IM rather than SC
- [ ] add hydrocortisone 50-100 mg to the syringe

Care of syringe driver and injection site

Routine	When things go wrong
Choice of infusion sites	*Infusion stopped or too slow*
Upper chest (intercostal plane)	Inflamed injection site?
Upper arm (outer aspect)	Cannula kinked?
Abdomen	Start button not pressed?
Thighs	Battery failure?
	If none of above true, the machine needs servicing
Each day	*Infusion too fast*
Examine site: change if inflamed	Check rate setting
Check rate	Check rate calculation
Press operation test button where applicable	
Fill new syringe	If both correct, the machine is faulty and needs servicing

---

Classification of Opioids

Opioids may be classified in a number of ways

- By efficacy (i.e. weak, strong)
- By chemical structure
- By receptor activity

Classification by chemical structure

Opium
standardized opium
papaveretum ('strong opium')

Naturally occurring
codeine
morphine
} extracted from opium

Semisynthetic
dihydrocodeine
oxycodone†
diamorphine*
hydromorphone†
oxymorphone†
nalbuphine
buprenorphine
} obtained by relatively simple structural modifications of the morphine, codeine or thebaine molecule

Synthetic
☐ *Morphinans*
   pentazocine
   levorphanol

☐ *Phenylpiperidines*
   pethidine/meperidine
   anileridine
   fentanyl

☐ *Diphenylpropylamines*
   dextropropoxyphene
   dipipanone*
   dextromoramide*
   methadone
} synthetic compounds with structural resemblance to the whole or to a part of the morphine molecule

Classification by receptor activity

Type	Definition	Example
Agonist	A drug which combines with a receptor and activates it, initiating the pharmacological response associated with that drug	morphine (mu agonist)
Antagonist	A drug which interferes with the action of an agonist; a 'pure' antagonist has minimal or no agonist activity	naloxone
Partial agonist	A drug which elicits less than maximal response from interaction with the receptor; if a partial agonist displaces a complete agonist, the result may be a decreased response	buprenorphine (mu agonist)
Mixed agonist-antagonist	A drug acting simultaneously on different receptor sub-types, with the potential for both agonist action on one or more types and antagonist action on one or more types; the agonist activity may be partial or complete	pentazocine (partial kappa agonist-mu antagonist)

■ The body contains multiple opioid receptors, e.g. mu, kappa, delta, sigma

■ An opioid can be an agonist at one or more receptors; likewise an antagonist. For example, morphine is mainly a mu agonist whereas pentazocine is a kappa agonist and a mu antagonist

■ Opioids differ in receptor affinity ('potency') and intrinsic activity ('efficacy')

■ An opioid with relatively low intrinsic activity cannot exert a full agonist effect at individual receptors and is termed a partial agonist

Opioid	Receptor	Receptor affinity	Intrinsic activity
morphine	mu	+ +	+ + + +
buprenorphine	mu	+ + + +	+ +

- Because of differences in receptor affinity and intrinsic activity, a range of interactions are possible when two opioids are given concurrently. For example, if morphine is occupying all the mu receptors and buprenorphine, a partial agonist with high receptor affinity, is administered, some of the morphine will be displaced. This will result in a reduced opioid effect. In other words, buprenorphine can antagonize by displacement of morphine. On the other hand, if morphine is occupying only a proportion of the mu receptors, administering buprenorphine will result in an enhanced opioid effect

- Kappa agonists tend also to cause psychotomimetic effects

- Because of the possibility of antagonism, it is best not to use mu agonists and kappa agonists concurrently

- Likewise, it is best not to mix partial and complete agonists

Buprenorphine

- A semisynthetic thebaine derivative with potent partial mu-agonist properties

- An alternative to oral morphine in the low-middle part of morphine's dose range

- In low doses, buprenorphine and morphine are probably additive in their effects; at high doses, antagonism by buprenorphine may occur

- Buprenorphine is available as a SL tablet*. Ingestion reduces bioavailability

- Needs to be given only q8h; to give more often will make life unnecessarily harder for the patient

- With daily doses of over 3 mg, patients may prefer to take fewer tablets more often, i.e. q6h

- Analgesic ceiling at a daily dose of 3-5 mg. This is equivalent to 180-300 mg of oral morphine

- Buprenorphine is *not* an alternative to codeine or dextropropoxyphene. Like morphine, it should be used when a weak opioid has failed

■ Assuming previous regular use of codeine or dextropropoxyphene, patients should start on 0.2 mg q8h with the advice that:

'If it is not more effective than your previous tablet take a further 0.2 mg after 1 hour, and 0.4 mg q8h after that.'

■ When changing to morphine, multiply total daily dose by 60. If pain previously poorly controlled, multiply by 100

■ Adverse effects need to be monitored as with morphine: nausea, vomiting, constipation, drowsiness

■ There is never need to prescribe both buprenorphine and morphine. Use one or the other; then unintended antagonism cannot occur

Radiation Therapy

Radiation should be considered whenever pain is caused directly or indirectly by an osseous metastasis or by nerve compression.

Single dose treatment, or short courses (2–4 fractions) are often possible, particularly in peripheral sites.

Radiation gives partial or complete relief in >90% of patients experiencing bone pain. Recalcification occurs in 80%. Radiation is usually inappropriate in patients with a very short life expectancy (<2 weeks).

Radiation therapy and symptom control	
Bone pain	
Compression	brachial plexus
	lumbosacral plexus
	cauda equina
	spinal cord
	brain
	superior vena caval obstruction
	porta hepatis
Malignant ulcer	superficial
	rectal
Blood loss	haemoptysis
	haematuria
	vaginal

Corticosteroids

Inclusion in the following list does *not* mean that a corticosteroid is the treatment of choice for any given indication.

General uses	*Specific uses*
To improve appetite	Hypercalcaemia
To enhance sense of	Incipient paraplegia
well-being	Carcinomatous neuromyopathy
To improve strength	Superior vena caval obstruction
	Carcinomatous lymphangitis
	Haemoptysis
	Obstruction:
	bronchus
	ureter
Pain relief	[intestine]
Raised intracranial	Pericardial effusion
pressure	Rectal discharge (give PR)
Nerve compression	Diaphoresis/sweating
Spinal cord compression	Hormone therapy
Metastatic arthralgia	To reduce radiation-induced
[Bone pain]	inflammation
	Leucoerythroblastic anaemia

Dexamethasone is a convenient drug to use, particularly when high doses are indicated. Because of cost, prednisolone is often preferred in the USA.

In the UK, dexamethasone is available in 0.5 mg and 2 mg tablets; in the USA, 0.5 mg, 0.75 mg, 1 mg, 1.5 mg, 2 mg, 4 mg and 6 mg tablets. The largest prednisolone tablet is 5 mg. (In some countries a 20 mg tablet is available).

Dexamethasone is 7 times more potent than prednisolone. Thus 2 mg of dexamethasone is approximately equivalent to 15 mg of prednisolone.

Generally, corticosteroids may be administered as a single morning dose. In patients receiving replacement therapy after pituitary or adrenal ablation, however, cortisone acetate is given b.i.d.

For most indications, dexamethasone is usually given in a dose of 4 mg initially, reducing to a maintenance dose of 2 mg after 10–14 days. The main exceptions are:

Indication	Initial dose	Maintenance dose
Nerve compression	4 mg b.i.d.	2–4 mg daily or tailed off
Raised intra-cranial pressure	4 mg b.–q.i.d.	variable
Spinal cord compression	6–8 mg q.i.d.	usually tailed off after radiation

Phenytoin enhances the metabolism of dexamethasone but not of prednisolone. If phenytoin and dexamethasone are prescribed concurrently, a higher dose of dexamethasone may be necessary.

Prescribe initially as 'a trial of therapy'. Unless definite improvement is seen after 7-10 days, the corticosteroid should be tailed off over 3–4 days.

The initial arbitrary dose should be reviewed in the light of benefits and unwanted effects. Sometimes, it is possible to discontinue treatment altogether.

Oral Candidiasis is a common unwanted effect. Ankle oedema and moonfacing less so. The latter may limit treatment, necessitating dose reduction or cessation of treatment.

Agitation, insomnia or a more florid psychiatric disturbance may be precipitated by corticosteroids. The use of diazepam at bedtime is sometimes indicated to counter agitation or insomnia.

Deafferentation Pain

Definition Nerve destruction pain

Synonym — dysaesthetic pain

Characteristics

■ Distribution — dermatomal if peripheral nerve; non-dermatomal if central

■ Quality — superficial burning or stinging discomfort. There may also be spontaneous stabbing/lancinating pain
An associated deep ache may relate to nerve compression (mixed compression-deafferentation pain) or be a variant manifestation of deafferentation

■ Associations — light touch or blowing exacerbates pain (allodynia). Unable to bear clothing against affected area.
Pinprick and temperature sensations are usually diminished
Sometimes there is numbness as well
Often receiving morphine with minimal or no effect, and exhausted because of pain-related insomnia

Management

■ Explanation
  □ 'Nerve damage pain'. 'Does not respond to pain-killers like aspirin and morphine'
  □ 'Need to phase out unhelpful medication'
  □ 'Need to start a tricyclic drug at bedtime'. 'Crucial to get a good night's sleep'

■ Medication
  □ tricyclic drug, e.g. amitriptyline, clomipramine, imipramine
  □ anticonvulsant, e.g. sodium valproate, carbamazepine
  □ local anaesthetic congener, e.g. flecainide, mexiletine
  □ corticosteroid (?), e.g. dexamethasone, prednisolone

Therapeutic Guidelines

Tricyclic drug

	Elderly frail/ outpatient	Younger patient/ inpatient
25 mg nocte	Week 1	Day 1
50 mg nocte	Week 2	Day 2–4
75 mg nocte	Week 3 + 4	Day 5–21
100 mg nocte	Week 5 + 6	Week 3 + 4
150 mg nocte	Week 7 + 8	Week 5 + 6

■ Clomipramine and imipramine cause less marked anticholinergic effects than amitriptyline and are to be preferred in the elderly and/or debilitated

■ Speed of increase depends on severity of the pain and on degree of supervision. Onset of relief unusual before day 4-5 and unlikely with only 25 mg

■ It is unusual to need more than 100 mg in cancer-related deafferentation pain.

■ Maximum dose is determined by the degree of relief and by unwanted effects. Unwanted effects are a common limiting factor.

Anticonvulsant

■ Sodium valproate has a long plasma half-life and is sedative. Given as a single dose nocte. In the younger patient start with 500 mg nocte; in the elderly 200 mg. Build up dose every 3–4 days to 1000–1500 mg. As cumulation will occur, it may be possible subsequently to reduce the dose

■ Many centres use carbamazepine. The dose of carbamazepine must be built up slowly (200 mg/week). When given with a tricyclic drug, the metabolism of *both drugs* is slowed down. Needs to be taken several times a day.

Local anaesthetic congener

■ Major disadvantage is the negative inotropic effect on the heart. *Should not be given to patients with evidence of cardiac failure*. A baseline ECG (electrocardiogram) is advisable to exclude conduction abnormalities that might be exacerbated.

- Central nervous system toxicity includes confusional symptoms, paraesthesiae, multifocal myoclonus, fitting and coma. A smaller dose is indicated in renal failure

- Flecainide is the drug of choice for deafferentation pain at some centres

- Start with flecainide 50 mg b.i.d. Increase to 100 mg b.i.d. after 3–4 days if there are no troublesome unwanted effects. If no benefit, increase to 150 mg b.i.d. after a further 7–10 days

- If successful, an attempt should be made to reduce the dose by one decrement after a further 1–2 weeks

- Flecainide should *not* be used in conjunction with a tricyclic drug because of an increased likelihood of cardiac arrhythmias. It may be used with an anticonvulsant

Corticosteroid

- Dexamethasone 4 mg b.i.d. *or* prednisolone 20–30 mg b.i.d. will have no effect in pure deafferentation pain but, in cancer, it may convert a mixed pain into a more opioid responsive nerve compression pain

Sympathetic Maintained Pain

Occasionally a cancer patient presents with an opioid resistant pain which is dependent on the integrity of the sympathetic nerves. In other words, a regional sympathetic nerve block relieves the pain.

As sympathetic fibres are efferent only, this is surprising. It is probable that some somatic afferent fibres associated with nociception travel with the sympathetic nerves.

Sympathetic maintained pain in cancer is similar to causalgia, a post-traumatic sympathetic maintained pain syndrome.

Assessment

The essential features are

- Pain (often burning)
- Sensory disorder
- Relief following sympathetic block

It is necessary to differentiate between the burning pain of deafferentation and the burning pain of a sympathetic maintained pain. This can be difficult as features are not constant and some are common to both conditions.

Superficial burning pain		
	Somatic deafferentation	Sympathetic maintained
Cause	nerve destruction	nerve irritation (?)
Pattern	dermatomal (if peripheral)	*non-dermatomal*
Concomitants		
stabbing pain	common	unusual
allodynia[1]	+	+/−
hyperpathia[1]	+/−	+/−
deep pressure	comforts	tender near joints (common)
pinprick	diminished (usually)	diminished (usually)
muscle atrophy	+	+/−
muscle fatigue	−	+/−
trophic changes	late	early[2]
limb temperature	normal/cold	usually colder[3]
Tricyclic drug	good relief (often)	little or no relief
Sympathetic block	no relief	partial or complete relief

1 See definitions on p. 39.
2 Trophic changes may affect skin, subcutaneous tissues and/or nails; may be atrophic (e.g. shiny taut skin, hair loss) or hypertrophic (e.g. hyperkeratosis).
3 If in doubt, temperature changes can be confirmed with a thermo-couple. Valid only if the pulses are equal in both the affected and normal limbs, and no history of deep venous thrombosis. In some patients the temperature may vary with warm episodes and sweating.

- May be radiographic evidence of osteoporosis and of hot spots on isotope bone scans; these may be mistaken for osteolytic metastases

- The distribution of sympathetic maintained pain does not correspond with the dermatomal pattern of the peripheral nerves. Instead it reflects the pattern of sympathetic vascular innervation

Arterial supply of the skin

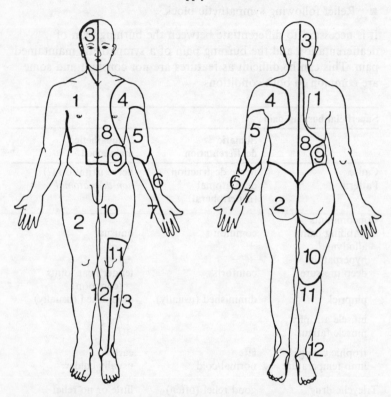

1 Subclavian artery = cervicothoracic trunk outflow = upper quadrant of the body
2 Iliac arteries = lumbar sympathetic outflow = lower quadrant of the body

3	Common carotid artery	4	Axillary artery
5	Brachial artery	6	Radial artery
7	Ulnar artery	8	Thoracic aorta
9	Abdominal aorta	10	Femoral artery
11	Popliteal artery	12	Posterior tibial artery
13	Anterior tibial artery		

(Reproduced from Gerbershagen HU 1979 Blocks with local anesthetics in the treatment of cancer pain. In: *Advances in Pain Research and Therapy Volume 2.* Edited by Bonica JJ & Ventafridda V. Raven Press, New York)

Treatment

If sympathetic maintained pain is suspected, arrangements should be made for the patient to have a diagnostic sympathetic block with local anaesthetic. This not only serves to confirm the diagnosis but also may give relief that outlasts the duration of action of the local anaesthetic.

A neurolytic block is worth considering at a later date for lower limb pain if symptoms return. Lumbar sympathectomy under radiographic control is a safe procedure with minimal unwanted effects.

Pain Terms (International Association for the Study of Pain)

Allodynia	Pain caused by a stimulus which does not normally provoke pain
Analgesia	Absence of pain in response to stimulation which would normally be painful
Central Pain	Pain associated with a lesion of the central nervous system (CNS)
Dysaesthesia	An unpleasant abnormal sensation, whether spontaneous or evoked
Hyperaesthesia	Increased sensitivity to stimulation
Hyperalgesia	An increased response to a stimulus which is normally painful
Hyperpathia	A painful syndrome characterized by increased reaction to a stimulus, especially a repetitive stimulus, *as well as an increased threshold.* [This latter feature results in a delayed onset. It tends to be poorly localized and outlasts the stimulus.]
Neuralgia	Pain in the distribution of a nerve
Neuropathy	A disturbance of function or pathological change in a nerve
Nociceptor	A receptor preferentially sensitive to a noxious stimulus or to a stimulus which would become noxious if prolonged
Noxious Stimulus	A noxious stimulus is one which is damaging to normal tissues
Pain	An unpleasant sensory and emotional experience associated with actual or potential tissue damage or described in terms of such damage
Pain Threshold	The least experience of pain which a subject can recognize
Pain Tolerance Level	The greatest level of pain which a subject is prepared to tolerate

3 ALIMENTARY SYMPTOMS

Halitosis	Heartburn
Dry mouth	Nausea and vomiting
Stomatitis	Antacids
Oral Candidiasis	Squashed stomach syndrome
Abnormal taste	Gastrointestinal obstruction
Failure to eat	Constipation
Cachexia	Faecal impaction
Dysphagia	Rectal discharge
Endo-oesophageal tube	Ascites

Halitosis

Definition   Unpleasant or foul smelling breath.

Causes

■ Septic putrefactive changes within the mouth, pharynx, nose, nasal sinuses or lungs

■ Severe infections

■ Gastric stagnation associated with gastric outflow obstruction

■ Smoking or ingestion of substances, such as garlic, onions, alcohol or paraldehyde, whose volatile products are excreted by the lungs or saliva

Treatment Possibilities

General

□ attention to oral and dental hygiene
□ adequate fluid intake
□ treatment of oral Candidiasis
□ use of mouthwashes

Oropharyngeal malignancy

- povidone-iodine mouthwash ⎫
- antibiotics ⎭ if infection present
- hydrogen peroxide (1%) gargles, especially on waking, after meals and bedtime; *or* cider and soda water in equal parts
- artificial saliva, if mouth excessively dry as a result of disease or irradiation (Glandosane*, Xerolube†, Saliva Substitute†)

Lung sepsis

- patient generally complains of abundant foul-smelling sputum
- may be abnormal physical signs in the thorax
- sputum should be sent for culture and an antibiotic prescribed, e.g. amoxycillin *or* chloramphenicol
- if diffuse pulmonary Candidiasis, prescribe ketoconazole 200 mg b.i.d. PO

Dry Mouth

Dryness of the mouth may be caused by diminished secretion of saliva, diseased buccal mucosa or by excessive evaporation of fluid from the buccal cavity.

Causes

Cancer
Anxiety
Depression
Hypercalcaemia
Replacement of salivary
  glands by cancer
Erosion of buccal mucosa

Anticancer treatment
Local radiation
Local radical surgery
Stomatitis associated
  with granulocytopenia

Drugs
Anticholinergics:
  antihistamines
  antiParkinsonians
  antispasmodics
  belladonna alkaloids
  neuroleptics
  tricyclics
Opioids (uncommon)
Diuretics
Oxygen (without humidification)

Debility
Mouth breathing
Dehydration
Infection:
  Candidiasis
  parotitis

Concurrent
Uncontrolled diabetes
Hyperthyroidism
Auto-immune disease
Amyloid
Sarcoid

Treatment Possibilities

■ Explanation

■ Enlist assistance of family and friends
                                        ■ Review drug
regimen

■ Meticulous mouth care every 2 hours
  □ mouthwashes:
      *effervescent mouthwash tablets** — containing peppermint
      oil, clove oil, spearmint, menthol, thymol and
      methylsalicylic acid in an effervescent base; when
      dissolved they make a palatable and refreshing
      mouthwash
      cetylpyridinium and alcohol (Merocet*, Cepacol†) — a
      cationic surfactant disinfectant
      hexetidine 0.1% (Oraldene*) — has weak antibacterial
      and antifungal activity

□ debridement of furred tongue:
use soft toothbrush and hydrogen peroxide 1% *or* cider and soda water (equal parts), *or* urea hydrogen peroxide† (Glyoxide)

■ Dietary advice
□ something in the mouth, e.g. pipe stem, chewing gum
□ strongly flavoured candy:
cinnamon
acid drops
lemon drops
Lifesavers†
□ pineapple chunks

■ Moisten mouth and lips
□ frequent mouth care
□ water by dropper
□ gauze bag containing ice placed between tongue and gums every 30 min
□ a room humidifier
□ frequent thin layer of petroleum jelly to lips (not a thick coating once a day)

■ Artificial salivas
□ Glandosane spray*; Xerolube spray†; Saliva Substitute†
□ Connecticut formulation:
methylcellulose 12 g
lemon essence 0.2 ml
water to 600 ml
Dilute with equal amount of water to 1200 ml, i.e. dispensed double strength to reduce cost
Need to use every hour to keep mouth well lubricated; administer by 1 ml dropper

■ Treat oral Candidiasis (see p. 46)

Stomatitis

Definition

A general term applied to diffuse inflammatory, erosive and ulcerative conditions affecting the mucous membranes lining the mouth.

Synonym — sore mouth

Pathogenesis

- Malnutrition
  - hypovitaminosis
  - anaemia
  - protein deficiency
- Altered immunity
- Drugs
  - cytotoxic
  - corticosteroids
  - antibiotics
- Infection
  - Candidiasis
  - aphthous ulcers
- Dry mouth

Treatment Possibilities

- Treat dry mouth (see p. 42)
- Modify drug regimen
- Treat Candidiasis (see p. 46)
- Treat aphthous ulcers

Drug treatment of aphthous ulcers

Antibiotics and antiseptics
tetracycline suspension
chlorhexidine gluconate gel (Corsodyl dental gel)

Inflammatory and immune suppression
hydrocortisone
triamcinolone acetonide
betamethasone-17-benzoate

- Symptomatic measures
  - choline salicylate* (Bonjela gel)
  - benzydamine* (Difflam)
  - sucralfate 1 g tablet — crush and spread around mouth
    with the tongue
  - local anaesthetics:
      lignocaine viscous 2%
      benzocaine (Merocaine*, Hurricaine†)
      dyclonine† (Diclone)
  - diphenhydramine† local application

Benzydamine hydrochloride — a NSAID which is absorbed through the skin and buccal mucosa; it also has a mild local anaesthetic action. Benzydamine gargle (15 ml) is of proven value in radiation-induced buccal mucositis. It may sting initially.

Diphenhydramine† in Kaopectate — comprises equal parts of diphenhydramine elixir† (12.5 mg/5 ml) and Kaopectate. The pectin in the Kaopectate is thought to help the diphenhydramine adhere to the mucosal surface. It is spread around the mouth with the tongue and then swallowed. Use up to 30 ml q2h.

Stomatitis cocktail (National Cancer Institute, USA) — comprises lignocaine viscous 2%, diphenhydramine elixir† 12.5 mg/5 ml), and Maalox (proprietary antacid) in equal parts. It is spread around the mouth with the tongue, held for 2 min and then spat out. Use up to 30 ml q2h.

Oral Candidiasis

Dry mouth, corticosteroids and bacterial antibiotics are common precipitating causes.

If using a topical fungal antibiotic, advise patient to remove and clean dentures before each dose. Failure to treat dentures may lead to failure to control Candidiasis.

At night, soak dentures in water containing nystatin (5 ml); *or* in diluted sodium hypochlorite solution* (Milton)

Most patients respond to a 10 day course. Some need continuous treatment.

Fungal Antibiotics

- Nystatin:
  - □ suspension (100 000 units/ml) 1-5 ml q4h
  - □ pastilles (100 000 units)
  - □ popsicles† (home-made) 5 ml of nystatin suspension mixed with cherry Kool-Aid†, freeze in ice tray with rounded cups

■ Ketoconazole 200 mg tablet daily
Take after food to reduce gastric irritation Acts systemically;
useful also for vaginal Candidiasis

■ Fluconazole* 50 mg capsule daily. Acts systemically. If
marked renal failure give on alternate days after third dose. In
contrast to ketoconazole, has negligible effect on P450-mediated
enzymes involved in the synthesis of adrenal corticosteroids,
progesterone, testosterone and oestrogens. Available in the USA
for HIV-positive patients on Compassionate Usage Program

■ Miconazole 125 mg/5 ml gel q.i.d. Administer by teaspoon
— the patient spreads it around the mouth with the tongue

Abnormal Taste

Many patients with advanced cancer experience a change in
taste sensation. This is not related to primary site, other
alimentary symptoms or prognosis.

Incidence
All cancer — 50%

Relevant Pathophysiology
This is largely presumptive.

■ Decreased sensitivity of taste buds

■ Decreased number of taste buds

■ Toxic dysfunction of taste buds

■ Nutritional deficiencies → altered sensation

■ Poor dental hygiene

Clinical Manifestations

■ Vague complaint that 'food does not taste right'
'Everything is tasteless'
'I have a metallic taste in my mouth'

■ Changes in threshold, e.g.
  □ high threshold for sweetness (sucrose)
  □ low threshold for sweetness (sucrose)
  □ low threshold for bitterness (urea)

Treatment Possibilities

- Reduce urea content of diet: eat white meats, eggs, dairy products

- Mask bitter taste of urea containing food
  - add wine and beer to soups and sauces
  - marinate chicken, fish, meat
  - use more and stronger seasonings
  - eat food cold or at room temperature
  - drink more liquids

- To help overcome general poor taste
  - tart foods (pickles, lemon juice, vinegar)
  - eat food which leaves its own taste (fresh fruit, hard candy)

- Dental check up

Failure To Eat

Whose problem is it? Patient or family?
It is natural for people close to death to lose interest in food and, to a lesser extent, in fluids. Before a natural disinterest is accepted as the main causal factor, reversible causes should be excluded.

Causes	Treatment possibilities
Fear of vomiting	Antiemetics
Unappetizing food	Choice of food *by patient*
Offered too much food	Small meals
Early satiation	Snacks between meals
Dehydration	Rehydrate
Constipation	Laxatives
Mouth discomfort	Mouth care (see p. 43)
Pain	Analgesics
Fatigue	Rest
Malodourous ulcer	Prevention of malodour
Biochemical:	
hypercalcaemia	Correction of hypercalcaemia
hyponatraemia	
uraemia	
Secondary to treatment:	
drugs	Modify drug regimen
irradiation	
chemotherapy	
Disease process	Trial of corticosteroids
Anxiety	Anxiolytic
Depression	Antidepressive

Therapeutic Guidelines

- Explanation

- Listen to the family's fears

- Discourage 'He must eat or he will die' syndrome
Emphasize that you are not too concerned whether or not the
patient gets a rounded diet:
'Don't feed him for the sake of science or for my sake'
'Just give him a little of what he fancies'
'I shall be happy even if he just takes fluids'
'After all, babies thrive on milk'
'His system is so sick, he cannot digest much food'

- Understand and be prepared to offer simple psychological
support to overcome the 'food as love' and 'but feeding him is
my job' syndromes

- A small helping looks better on a smaller plate — do not
use large dinner plates

- Food available when *patient* hungry — a microwave oven
helps to achieve this

- Offer specific dietary advice

- Eating is a social habit — we eat better at a table and
when dressed

- Prevention of malodour (see p. 160)

- Appetite stimulants
  □ corticosteroid, e.g:
      prednisolone 10–30 mg daily *or*
      dexamethasone 2–4 mg daily
  □ amitriptyline 25–50 mg nocte
  □ cyproheptadine 4 mg t.i.d.

Cachexia

Definition   Severe wasting.

Cachexia in cancer patients is not directly correlated with food
intake or the site, histological type or stage of the tumour. It may
antedate the clinical diagnosis and can occur with a very small
primary neoplasm.

Incidence

All cancer — 30% (range 10–75%)
Highest incidence in gastrointestinal and bronchogenic
carcinoma

Causes

Anorexia → deficient food intake
Vomiting
Diarrhoea
Malabsorption
Increased metabolic rate → increased energy expenditure
Abnormal host metabolism of:
   protein
   carbohydrate
   fat
   hormones
   water
   electrolytes
Nitrogen trap by the tumour
Tumour products (e.g. cachectin)
Debilitating effect of treatment:
   surgery
   radiation
   chemotherapy
Ulceration ⎫
Haemorrhage ⎬ excessive loss of body protein

Clinical Manifestations

- Anorexia and early satiation

- Looks ill (weight loss)

- Muscle weakness

- Lethargy

- Pallor (anaemia)

- Oedema (hypoalbuminaemia)

- Loss of body protein and fat

- Electrolyte disturbances

Complications and Consequences

- Altered appearance engenders fear and isolation

- Difficulty in social and family relationships

- Role change within the family
- Ill-fitting clothes increase sense of loss and displacement
- Loose dentures cause pain and eating difficulties
- Pressure sores

Therapeutic Considerations

- Because of the greatly increased metabolic rate, aggressive dietary supplementation (nasogastric tube, IV hyperalimentation) is of little value in reversing cachexia in the dying patient

- Therapeutic efforts are better directed towards ameliorating the social consequences and physical complications

- Dental relining done at the bedside will last 3 months; it restores chewing abilities and improves facial appearance

- An old photo from before the weight loss will help the new caregivers recognize the essential humanness of the emaciated cachectic individual

- Equally, new photos taken of the emaciated patient with the family and friends will help to legitimize the value of this 'different' person, emphasizing that he still occupies a place in the world

- If it can be afforded, a new set of well fitting clothes pays handsome dividends in enhanced self-esteem

- Patient and family need education about the new bony prominences and the importance of skin care (see p. 147)

- Explain to the family
  - how they can assist the fickle appetite (see p. 48)
  - that the patient will be satisfied with less intake, and that this is normal

- Avoid routine weighing of the patient

- The loan of items designed to enhance personal independence in the face of weakness, e.g. wheelchair, ramps, raised toilet seat, commode, hospital bed, walking frame, mat for the bathtub

Dysphagia

Definition   Difficulty in swallowing.

Relevant Physiology

There are three stages of swallowing

- Buccal — passage of bolus to the back of the throat
- Pharyngeal — voluntary initiation of swallowing reflex
- Oesophageal — involuntary reflex peristalsis

Two basic processes cause dysphagia

- Mechanical obstruction
- Neuromuscular defects

Assessment

- Distinguish from odynophagia (painful swallowing)
- Obstructing lesions usually produce dysphagia for solids
initially, with later progression to liquids

- Neuromuscular disorders cause dysphagia for both solids and
liquids about the same time.

Causes

Cancer	Treatment
Mass lesion in mouth, pharynx or oesophagus	Surgery: lingual buccal
Linear infiltration of pharyngo-oesophageal wall→ damage to nerve plexus	Post-radiation fibrosis: difficulty in opening mouth and moving tongue
External compression (mediastinal mass)	prolonged oesophageal transit oesophageal strictures
Perineural tumour spread (vagus and sympathetic chain)	Upward displacement of endo-oesophageal tube
Tumour spread to base of skull (lower cranial nerve palsies)	
Non-metastatic neuromuscular dysfunction	
Hypercalcaemia	
Anxiety → oesophageal spasm	**Debility**
	Pharyngo-oesophageal Candidiasis
Concurrent	Excessive drowsiness and disinterest
Benign oesophageal stricture	Extreme weakness (patient moribund)

Treatment Possibilities

- Explanation

- Agreement between patient, family and staff about treatment potential and feeding goals

- Dietary advice
  - recommend suitable soft food cookbooks
  - use of liquidizer/blenderizer
  - cold sour cream (by the spoonful)

- Attempt to retard lumen constriction
  - trial of corticosteroids
  - radiation therapy
  - laser treatment
  - intermittent bouginage with blunt tipped bougie

- Feeding tubes
  - Clinifeed* or Dobhoff enteric tube†
    transnasal placement by doctor on ward possible if
    oesophageal lumen > 1 cm
  - Celestin indwelling endo-oesophageal tube
    plastic, placed by surgeon with upper abdominal incision
    or via flexible fibreoptic oesophagoscope; patient able to
    eat semisolid diet

- Reduction of saliva if total obstruction produces sialorrhoea
  and drooling
  - antisialogogues
    propantheline
    tricyclic drug   }
    piperazine phenothiazine } anticholinergics
    belladonna alkaloid   }
  - irradiation of salivary glands
    400–1000 cGy for temporary reduction in secretion

Endo-Oesophageal Tube

An indwelling flexible endo-oesophageal tube (e.g. Celestin) can
be used to maintain a passage for fluid and food through a
narrowed portion of the oesophagus and/or gastro-oesophageal
junction. The upper end is broader in diameter; this impedes

downward displacement, and serves as a funnel for ingested matter.

The tube is introduced by a surgeon through an upper abdominal incision or via a fibreoptic oesophagoscope.

Indications for Use

■ Marked dysphagia for semisolids including liquidized/blenderized foods

■ Patient relatively independent and active. A tube is not indicated in moribund patients

Postoperative Management

■ Nursed with shoulders elevated on 2–3 pillows to prevent reflux of gastric contents

■ Ascertain position of the tube by Gastrografin swallow 3–4 days after operation

■ Begin with fluid diet but change after 1–2 days to a semisolid one. Solids by postoperative day 6–7

■ *Patient must be trained to chew food twice as long as normal*

■ Sips of a carbonated drink are taken frequently during and after every meal, however small

This advice may need to be modified in patients with squashed stomach or small stomach syndrome.

■ *The following foods should be avoided completely*
   □ *all forms of fish*
   □ *hard boiled eggs*
   □ *oranges and other pithy fruit*

The tube rarely gets blocked if instructions are carefully followed by the patient. In case of blockage, limit to small amounts of water and, every half hour, sips of dilute hydrogen peroxide. This usually clears the tube within 3–4 h.

■ Radiotherapy does not affect the tube

Advice to Patient and Family

[Modified from Thoracic Surgical Unit, Oxford]

In addition to verbal and visual explanation about the tube, the following written advice should be given to each patient:

A plastic tube has been put into your gullet to help you get your food down more easily

Unfortunately the tube tends to limit what you can eat and may become blocked if you do not *chew* your food *very thoroughly* before swallowing it

You should avoid *fish, hard boiled eggs, orange pulp*

Mince all meat unless soft and easily chewed

Peas should be pureed or carefully chewed

Sip a *fizzy* drink during each meal

If the tube becomes blocked and does not clear with a slow fizzy drink, contact your doctor

---

Foods to enjoy

All drinks	Mashed potatoes
Alcohol	Liquidized vegetables
	Liquidized fruits
Porridge	Mashed banana
Lightly boiled egg	Milk puddings
	Instant Whip
Minced meat and chicken	Angel Delight
Minced bacon and ham	Jelly and blancmange
Liquidized fish	Custard
Dry crustless bread and butter	Sponge cake
Jams, marmalade and jellies	Crumbly (not flaky) biscuits/ cookies
Finely grated cheese	

Do not eat

Lumpy and stringy foods and fruit	Chunks of cheese
Poached, fried or hard boiled egg	Chips and fried potatoes
	Raw vegetables unless liquidized
Fish unless liquidized	
Other sea food	Dumplings and stodgy puddings
Fresh bread and toast	Scones and cakes

Never take tablets unless crushed or dissolved

Heartburn

Definition

A burning retrosternal discomfort which tends to radiate upwards. It is usually caused by the reflux of acidic gastric contents into the oesophagus.

Associated Symptoms

- Regurgitation

- Odynophagia (painful swallowing) — a retrosternal ache

- Dysphagia — transient, for solid foods only

- Water brash

- Intermittent cough or wheezing

- Weakness secondary to bleeding

Pathophysiology

A 5 cm length of distal oesophagus functions as a high pressure zone (normally 10–12 mmHg) to prevent reflux. This is known as the lower oesophageal sphincter (LES).

The LES relaxes with swallowing. Its tone increases when the stomach is filled.

Reflux occurs when the LES fails to present an effective barrier.

Factors Decreasing the Competence of LES

Dietary	Drugs
Alcohol	Anticholinergics
Chocolate	Calcium channel blockers
Fat	Diazepam
Carminatives:	Nitrates and nitrites
peppermint	Oestrogens
anise	Pethidine/meperidine
dill	Theophylline
Carbonated beverages	
Aerophagic habits:	Mechanical
chewing gum	Constricting abdominal garments
sucking hard candy	Obesity
Oversized meals	Ascites
	Sleeping flat
Smoking (nicotine)	

Treatment Possibilities

- Explanation

- Diet — avoid precipitating factors

- Stop smoking

- Mechanical factors
  - avoid:
    - constricting garments
    - recumbency after eating
  - suggest:
    - elevate head of bed — 10 cm is sufficient
    - consider paracentesis
    - weight loss for obese

- Increase LES pressure
  - metoclopramide, domperidone*
  - bethanechol (a cholinergic drug)
    this is not often symptomatically effective and may increase gastric acid secretion

- Reduce gastric acid
  - antacids
  - alginate containing antacid
  - H$_2$ receptor blockers:
    - cimetidine
    - ranitidine

Occasional heartburn usually responds promptly to antacids.

Anticholinergic therapy has no place in the therapy of heartburn; it delays gastric emptying and lowers LES pressure.

Nausea and Vomiting

Definitions

Nausea

An unpleasant sensation associated with the upper gastrointestinal tract, often accompanied by an urge to vomit.

Retching

Rhythmic, laboured, spasmodic movements of the diaphragm and abdominal muscles, usually occurring in the presence of nausea. These movements may precede bouts of vomiting or alternate with them.

Vomiting

The forceful expulsion of gastrointestinal contents through the mouth.

Relevant Physiology

Vomiting is controlled by the vomiting centre in the medullary reticular formation. Vomiting is induced when input from other areas reaches the vomiting centre, notably the chemoreceptor trigger zone in the floor of the fourth ventricle:

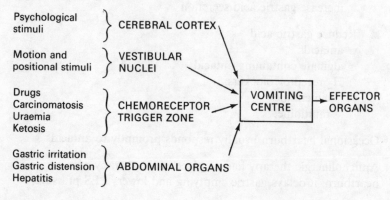

Assessment

■ Is the patient vomiting?
Exclude expectoration, regurgitation

■ Check fundi for papilloedema
Note: absence does not exclude raised intracranial pressure

■ Examine abdomen

■ Do rectal examination if impaction a possibility

- Consider checking
  - plasma urea and electrolytes
  - plasma calcium and albumin
  - plasma carbamazepine
  - plasma digoxin
- Review drug regimen

Causes

Cancer	Treatment
Irritation of upper gastrointestinal tract	Radiotherapy
	Chemotherapy
Blood in stomach	Drugs:
Gastrointestinal obstruction	antibiotics
	aspirin
Constipation	carbamazepine
Hepatomegaly	corticosteroids
Raised intracranial pressure	digoxin
	iron
Cough	irritant mucolytics (expectorants)
Pain	NSAID
Anxiety	oestrogens
Cancer toxicity	opioids
Hypercalcaemia	theophyllines
Hyponatraemia	
Uraemia	
	Concurrent
	Alcohol gastritis
	Cough
	Infection
	Peptic ulcer
	Uraemia

Treatment Possibilities

- Non drug measures include
  - a calm, reassuring environment, away from the sight and smell of food
  - small frequent feedings, e.g. 2–3 mouthfuls
  - avoid exposure to foods that precipitate nausea. This may mean transferring the patient to a single room

- If obstructed see p. 65

- Correct reversible causes
  - cough
  - constipation
  - raised intracranial pressure
  - hypercalcaemia

■ Use dispersible aspirin* *or* choline salicylate† (Arthropan) in place of standard aspirin

■ Consider stopping gastric irritant drugs
  □ antibiotic
  □ corticosteroid
  □ irritant mucolytic
  □ NSAID

Or prescribe an antacid or H_2 receptor blocker concurrently

■ Prescribe an appropriate antiemetic. Choice depends on
  □ cause of vomiting
  □ consideration of neurotransmitter receptor site affinity
  □ availability of oral/rectal/parenteral preparations

Antiemetic receptor site affinities

Drug group	Chemoreceptor trigger zone	Vomiting centre, Vestibular nuclei	
	Dopamine (D_2)	Muscarinic cholinergic	Histamine (H_1)
Anticholinergic			
hyoscine	0	+ + +	0
H_1 antihistamine			
diphenhydramine†	0	+	+ +
promethazine	+	+ +	+ + +
Neuroleptic			
fluphenazine	+ + +	+	+ +
prochlorperazine	+ +	0	+
chlorpromazine	+ +	+	+ +
droperidol	+ + +	0	0
haloperidol	+ + +	0	0
Gastrokinetic			
metoclopramide	+	0	0
Tricyclic			
amitriptyline	+	+ + +	+ + +
nortriptyline	+	+ +	+ +

Pharmacological activity: 0 = none or insignificant; + = slight;
+ + = moderate; + + + = marked. (Modified from Peroutka SJ & Snyder SH 1982 *Lancet* i: 658–9)

■ Corticosteroids, e.g. dexamethasone, methylprednisolone are of proven benefit in cisplatin-induced vomiting and are used in conjunction with high-dose metoclopramide IV and diazepam *or* lorazepam PO

- Cannabinoids and benzodiazepines exert an antiemetic effect mediated by the cerebral cortex
  - cannabinoids — dronabinol (THC), nabilone
  - benzodiazepines — lorazepam, diazepam

- H_1 antihistamine antiemetics include
  - cyclizine
  - meclozine
  - dimenhydrinate

Choice of Antiemetics

Cause of nausea and vomiting	Antiemetic of choice	Comment
Drug induced	haloperidol 1.5 mg nocte *or* fluphenazine 1 mg b.i.d.	Unwanted effects unusual at lower dose
Radiotherapy		
Chemotherapy		
Metabolic uraemia hypercalcaemia	haloperidol 5–20 mg/day *or* fluphenazine 2 mg b.-t.i.d.	Anticholinergic effects; may cause drowsiness
Raised intracranial pressure	cyclizine 50 mg b.-t.i.d. *or* meclozine† 25 mg b.-t.i.d.	Anticholinergic effects; may cause drowsiness
Intestinal obstruction		
Oesophageal reflux	metoclopramide 10–20 mg t.-q.i.d. *or* domperidone* 10–20 mg t.-q.i.d.	No anticholinergic effects
Delayed gastric emptying		
Gastric irritation by drug	treat gastritis change medication	May occur with NSAID and corticosteroids

Therapeutic Considerations

- Drug therapy is more successful if given prophylactically

- Suppositories and injections may be necessary to break a vicious circle

- At least 24 h of parenteral treatment should be given
  - if patient vomits back just after food or medicines

□ if patient vomits more than once every 8 h
(8 h = 1 nursing shift)

■ If the patient is the household cook, someone else may have
to take on this role

Antacids

Definition

Substances taken by mouth to neutralize gastric acid.

Classification

General antacids

□ sodium bicarbonate
□ magnesium salts
□ aluminium hydroxide
□ hydrotalcite (magnesium aluminium carbonate)
□ calcium carbonate

Proprietary preparations

Usually contain a mixture of magnesium and aluminium so as to
neutralize effect of bowels. May also contain sodium bicarbonate.

Modern developments

□ antiflatulents:
Asilone*
Maalox Plus
Mylanta†
to ease flatulence, distension, postprandial pain
□ alginic acid:
Gaviscon
Topal*
to prevent oesophageal reflux pain
□ bile salt binding agent:
hydrotalcite (Altacite*)
□ oxethazaine (a local anaesthetic in Mucaine*) to relieve
oesophageal pain

Precautions

■ Regular use of sodium bicarbonate may cause sodium loading and metabolic alkalosis

■ Regular use of calcium carbonate may cause hypercalcaemia, especially if taken with sodium bicarbonate

■ Magnesium salts → diarrhoea
Aluminium hydroxide → constipation

■ Many antacids contain sodium. This may be important in patients suffering from hypertension or cardiac failure

Preparation	Sodium content mmol(mEq)/10 ml
Liquid Gaviscon	6.3
Magnesium Trisilicate Mixture BP*	6.3
Aluminium Hydroxide Gel BP*	1.0
Mucaine* ⎫	0.6
Maalox ⎭	
Mylanta†	0.4
Asilone*	0.1

■ Aluminium hydroxide binds dietary phosphate. Of benefit in patients with hyperphosphataemia (in renal failure). Long-term complications of phosphate depletion and osteomalacia are not usually relevant in terminal care

■ Gaviscon needs both *acid* and *air bubbles* to produce an effective low density 'flotation cushion'

It may be less effective if used with an H_2 receptor blocker (reduces acid) and/or an antiflatulent (reduces bubbles).

Therapeutic Considerations

■ A 20 ml dose of most antacids q2h will reduce gastric acidity by up to 50%. H_2 receptor blockers have a similar effect during the day but cause greater nocturnal inhibition (⅔ compared with ⅓)

■ When fasting, conventional doses act for 20–40 min

■ A 20 ml dose 1 h after a meal neutralizes acid for 2 h

■ Except sodium bicarbonate, antacids delay gastric emptying

■ Some antacids contain *peppermint oil*. This helps eructation by decreasing the tone of the lower oesophageal sphincter. The mint flavour may, however, be a limiting factor in treatment

■ Most tablets feel gritty when sucked; this too may be a limiting factor

■ Antacids containing barbiturates and/or anticholinergic agents are *not* recommended

■ Cheapest preparations are:

Magnesium trisilicate BP* ⎱ may be given alone
Aluminium hydroxide Gel BP* ⎰ or in equal parts
Proportions may be varied if an equal parts mixture causes diarrhoea or constipation.

■ Alternative approaches

Drug	Action
metoclopramide ⎱ domperidone* ⎰	Hasten gastric emptying, tighten lower oesophageal sphincter
ranitidine (Zantac) ⎱ cimetidine (Tagamet)[1] ⎰	H$_2$ receptor blockers — reduce acid production

[1] Multiple drug interactions; much less with ranitidine

Squashed Stomach Syndrome

Definition

Dyspeptic symptoms associated with the inability of stomach to distend normally because of hepatomegaly or upper abdominal tumour. Similar symptoms may be seen with carcinoma of stomach, linitis plastica or postgastrectomy (small stomach syndrome).

Symptoms

■ Early satiation

■ Epigastric fullness

■ Epigastric discomfort/pain

■ Flatulence

■ Hiccup

■ Nausea

■ Vomiting (especially postprandial)

■ Heartburn

Treatment

- Explanation

- Dietary advice

- Antiflatulent (e.g. Asilone*, Maalox Plus 10 ml *after* meals and bedtime)

- Metoclopramide after meals and bedtime; or q4h with morphine

Gastrointestinal Obstruction

Definition

The impedance of forward propulsion of gastrointestinal contents as a result of an organic occlusion or the lack of normal propulsive activity or both — may be partial or complete

Symptoms vary according to the level of obstruction. Vomiting is most troublesome with more proximal obstruction, sometimes with little or no distension. Distension is also limited in patients with multiple small intestinal obstructions.

Assessment

With the help of previous laparotomy findings, plain abdominal X-rays, decide if the obstruction is in the large bowel, small bowel or pyloro-duodenum, and whether partial or complete.

Causes

Cancer	*Treatment*
Occlusive	Drugs
Non-occlusive (pseudo-obstruction):	Postoperative adhesions
intestinal linitis plastica	Post-radiation fibrosis
retroperitoneal neuropathy	
	Debility
	Faecal impaction

Drugs used in palliative care contributing to obstruction

- Action on smooth muscle
  - □ opioids

  These cause hypersegmentation of the bowel

- Anticholinergic drugs
  - □ antihistamines
  - □ belladonna alkaloids
  - □ neuroleptics
  - □ tricyclics

  These interfere with parasympathetic nerve transmission

- Paralytic ileus
  - □ anticoagulants

  The result of multiple intramural haemorrhages

- Mesenteric vascular occlusion
  - □ corticosteroids

Surgical Management

Surgical intervention should be considered if the following criteria are fulfilled

- If patient's general condition is good, i.e. independent and active with good previous symptom control

- Previous laparotomy findings do not preclude the prospect of successful intervention

- An easily reversible cause seems likely, e.g. postoperative adhesions or a single discrete neoplastic obstruction

- Patients willing to have surgery

In other circumstances, management should be non-surgical.

Medical Management

'Drip and Suck' (IV infusion + nasogastric suction) should be viewed as a preliminary to operative intervention, or a short-term expedient while a decision is taken concerning surgery. Such treatment does not form part of the continuing medical management of irreversible bowel obstruction in the patient with terminal cancer.

Constipation

Definition

Infrequent motions associated with difficulty of defaecation.

Normal Pattern of Defaecation

5–7/week 75%
$\left.\begin{array}{l} <3/\text{week} \\ >3/\text{day} \end{array}\right\}$ 1%

Complications of constipation

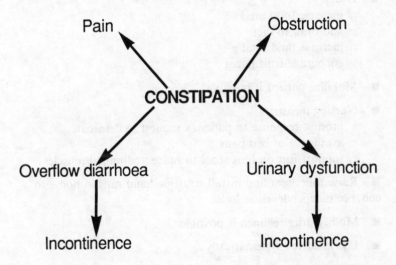

Causes

Cancer and debility	Drugs
Inactivity	Opioids
Poor nutrition:	Anticholinergics:
decreased intake	antihistaminic antiemetics
low residue diet	NSAID
Poor fluid intake	phenothiazines
Dehydration:	tricyclics
vomiting	
polyuria	Biochemical
fever	Hypercalcaemia
Weakness	Hypokalaemia
Inability to reach toilet	
when urge to defaecate	

Treatment Possibilities

- Diet
  - □ increase food intake
  - □ add bran to diet
  - □ increase fluid intake
  - □ encourage fruit juices

- Mobilize patient if possible

- Nursing measures
  - □ prompt response to patient's request to defaecate
  - □ avoidance of bed pans
  - □ support feet on foot stool to brace abdominal muscles

- Raise toilet seat and install strategic hand rails in home to enhance independence at toilet

- Modify drug regimen if possible

- Use laxatives systematically

- Rectal measures
  - □ suppositories
  - □ enemas
  - □ manual removals

Guidelines for management of opioid-induced constipation

Ask about the patient's usual bowel habit and use of laxatives

Do rectal examination if you suspect faecal impaction or if there is diarrhoea/faecal incontinence (to exclude impaction with overflow)

Record bowel motions each day in a 'Bowel Book'

Encourage fluids generally, fruit juice, fruit and bran

Prescribe prophylactically: co-danthrusate* 1 capsule nocte *or* casanthranol 30 mg with docusate 100 mg (Peri-Colace†) 1 capsule b.i.d.

If already constipated: co-danthrusate* 2 capsules nocte *or* Peri-Colace† 2 capsules b.i.d.

Adjust every few days according to results, up to 3 capsules q.i.d.

If necessary, 'uncork' with the help of bisacodyl (Dulcolax) 10 mg suppository + glycerine suppository

If suppositories are ineffective, administer a high phosphate enema (Fleets†) followed by a soap enema if no result

If the maximum dose of co-danthrusate* *or* Peri-Colace† is ineffective, reduce by half and add an osmotic laxative ('small bowel flusher'), e.g. lactulose 30 ml b.i.d.

If co-danthrusate* *or* Peri-Colace† causes abdominal cramps divide daily dose or change to a small bowel flusher, e.g. lactulose syrup 20–40 ml daily-t.i.d.

Lactulose may be preferable in patients with a history of irritable bowel syndrome (spastic colon) or of cramps with contact laxative ('peristaltic stimulants'), e.g. senna

Sometimes it is appropriate to optimize a patient's exisiting bowel regimen, rather than change automatically to co-danthrusate* *or* Peri-Colace†

Classification of laxatives

Bulk-forming drugs (dietary fibre)
Bran
Methylcellulose (Celevac*, Cologel*, Cellothyl†)
Mucilloids:
  psyllium (Metamucil)
  ispaghula (Isogel*, Fybogel*, Regulan*)
  sterculia (Normacol*)

Lubricants
Liquid paraffin* (mineral oil†)

Salines
Magnesium salts
Sodium sulphate
Sodium phosphate

Osmotic agents ('small bowel flushers')
Lactulose (Duphalac, Cephulac†, Chronulac†) Sorbitol (30–70%)
Mannitol (20%)

Contact laxatives ('peristaltic stimulants')
1 *Small and large bowel*
   Bile salts
   Castor oil (ricinoleic acid)　}　also *surface wetting agents*
   Docusate　　　　　　　　　　　　('faecal softeners')

2 *Mainly large bowel*
   Polyphenolics　　　　　　　　phenolphthalein
   　　　　　　　　　　　　　　　bisacodyl
   　　　　　　　　　　　　　　　sodium picosulphate
   Synthetic anthracene　　　　danthron*

3 *Large bowel only*
   Natural anthracenes　　　　　senna
   　　　　　　　　　　　　　　　casanthranol†
   　　　　　　　　　　　　　　　cascara†

Composition of laxatives (UK)

Co-danthrusate

capsule	danthron 50 mg & docusate 60 mg

Dioctyl

syrup (5 ml)	docusate 50 mg
tablet	docusate 100 mg

Senokot

tablet	sennoside B 7.5 mg

Dulcolax

tablet	bisacodyl 5 mg
suppository	bisacodyl 10 mg

Duphalac

syrup (5 ml)	lactulose 3.35 g

Magnesium salts

Milk of magnesia suspension (5 ml)	magnesium hydroxide 350 mg
Liquid paraffin and magnesium hydroxide emulsion BP (10 ml) (equivalent to 6% magnesium hydroxide)	magnesium hydroxide mixture BP 7.5 ml & liquid paraffin 2.5 ml
Epsom salts (crystals; 5 ml)	magnesium sulphate 4 g

Bulk forming drugs

Fybogel (sachet)	ispaghula husk 3.5 g
Normacol standard granules	sterculia 6.2g/10 g & frangula 800 mg/10 g
Normacol granules	sterculia 6.2g/10 g
Cologel liquid (/5 ml)	methylcellulose 450 mg
Celevac tablet	methylcellulose 500 mg
granules	methylcellulose 6.4 g/10 g

Composition of laxatives (USA)

Peri-Colace
capsule	casanthranol 30 mg & docusate 100 mg
solution (5 ml)	casanthranol 10 mg & docusate 20 mg

Colace
capsule	docusate 50 mg; 100 mg
solution (5 ml)	docusate 50 mg

Senokot
tablet	sennoside B 7.5 mg

Dulcolax
tablet	bisacodyl 5 mg
suppository	bisacodyl 10 mg

Milk of magnesia
suspension (5 ml)	magnesium hydroxide 350 mg
concentrate (5 ml)	magnesium hydroxide 1050 mg

Magnesium citrate
solution (10 oz)	magnesium citrate 17.45 g

Cascara sagrada and milk of magnesia
suspension (5 ml)	magnesium hydroxide 350 mg in cascara sagrada

Metamucil
powder packets	psyllium mucilloid 5 g/10 g & dextrose 5 g/10 g

Faecal Impaction

Definition

Lodging of faeces, most commonly in the rectum or descending colon but can occur as far back as the caecum.

Pathophysiology

Incomplete evacuation leads to accumulation of faeces in the rectum and/or colon. Fluid continues to be absorbed from the faeces as long as they remain in contact with the bowel mucosa. The faeces tend to become very firm.

Additional faecal material increases the size of the mass so that it is physically unable to pass through the anal sphincter.

Sometimes a soft impaction occurs. This is more likely if the impaction occurs despite the use of a bulk-forming drug or surface wetting agent.

Bacterial liquefaction of more proximal faeces may result in 'overflow' diarrhoea or faecal leakage.

Symptoms

- Complete cessation of faecal evacuation *or* frequent passage of small watery faeces *or* rectal discharge

- Abdominal distension (sometimes)

- Nausea and vomiting

- Abdominal colic (sometimes)

- Spasmodic rectal pain (occasional)

- Confusion, restlessness

Causes

Organic	*Drugs*
Tumour blocking passage	Aluminium antacids
of solid faeces	Anticholinergics
Anal stricture	Barium
	Opioids

General
Debility
Being bedfast
Mental impairment

Examination

There is usually a hard faecal mass in the rectum, *though an empty rectum does not rule out impaction.*

If the impaction is higher in the colon a faecal mass may be palpable in the abdomen. A faecal abdominal mass is non-tender, movable and usually indents.

Avoid oral barium if likelihood of an impaction exists.

Therapeutic Guidelines

Soft

- Bisacodyl suppository daily till negative response

- Contact with rectal mucosa is essential for absorption

- If mucosal contact impossible, use the oral route, though this has a less rapid effect

Hard

- Consider olive oil retention enema (120 ml) overnight, as a preliminary measure

- Consider premedication with IV midazolam *or* diazepam (see p. 115)

- Disrupt impaction in rectum by careful finger manipulation, and remove piece-meal if possible

- Follow by high instillation of Fletcher's arachis oil enema (if overnight olive oil enema not used)

- Rectal contents may be further softened by a retention enema of docusate 300 mg in 100 ml (use diluted oral syrup)

- Follow by a high enema
  - □ high phosphate enema *or*
  - □ isotonic saline ± soap enema
  Use an 18″ plastic catheter attached to enema giving set

- Institute measures to prevent recurrence

Rectal Discharge

Causes

- Haemorrhoids

- Faecal impaction

- Tumour

- Radiation proctitis

- Ileo-rectal, colo-rectal, recto-vesical fistula

Symptoms

- Discharge
- Maceration
- Pruritus
- Malodour

Treatment Possibilities

Correct or modify cause

- Faecal disimpaction (see p. 76)
- Reduce tumour size
  - radiation therapy
  - fulguration (surgical diathermy)
  - transanal resection
  - laser treatment
- Reduce peri-tumour or post-radiation inflammation
  - prednisolone suppositories (Predsol) 1 b.i.d.
  - prednisolone retention enema (Predsol) every 2–3 days

Alleviation of secondary symptoms

- Protection of skin of perineum and genitalia
  - do not use toilet paper
  - wash anal area with a soft cloth after each bowel movement and as necessary according to discharge
  - use water only — no soap
  - pat dry with soft cloth
  - if skin is unbroken (no stinging) apply methylated spirits *or* witch-hazel (Tucks†) and allow to dry
  - apply zinc stearate *or* other fine bland powder, eg. Johnson's baby powder
  - if inflamed use clioquinol (Vioform)-hydrocortisone cream, *or* hydrocortisone 0.25% spray† for 48 h
  - avoid ointments and creams to perineum and genitalia
  - if above measures do not keep the area dry, protect intact skin with zinc oxide paste
  - monitor carefully for tiny blisters suggestive of fungal infection; treat with clotrimazole 1% solution
  - tape buttocks apart if the patient finds this beneficial
  - use cotton underclothes and change at least daily
- Control pruritus

If anal hygiene fails to relieve, use sedative anti-pruritic drugs

Ascites

Definition

Excessive serous fluid in the peritoneal cavity.

Pathogenesis

- Usually associated with peritoneal metastases
- Subphrenic lymphatics become blocked by tumour infiltration
- Fluid exuded by peritoneum, possibly as a result of tumour-related vasoactive products
- Raised plasma renin concentration, possibly the result of a reduced extracellular blood volume, causes sodium retention

Clinical Features

- Abdominal distension, discomfort, pain
- Inability to sit upright
- Squashed stomach syndrome
- Lower oesophageal syndrome
- Nausea and vomiting
- Leg oedema
- Dyspnoea

Treatment Possibilities

- Chemotherapy
  - systematic
  - intraperitoneal
- Immunostimulation
  - systemic
  - intraperitoneal

■ Diuretics

Day	Spironolactone	Bumetanide	(Frusemide)
1	200 mg daily	1 mg	(60 mg)
4	200 mg b.i.d.	2 mg	(120 mg)
7	200 mg b.i.d.	2 mg + 2 mg	(120 mg + 120 mg)

Failure with diuretic therapy relates to
  □ therapeutic impatience
  □ too small a dose of spironolactone
  □ too small a dose of a loop diuretic

■ Paracentesis: a useful emergency measure in a distressed patient with a tense painful abdomen. Remove 2 L rapidly, then 5–6 L in 12 h

■ Peritoneovenous shunt: a useful option in a patient who is relatively well but cannot tolerate diuretic therapy

4 NEUROPSYCHOLOGICAL SYMPTOMS

Wakeful nights	Spinal cord compression
Weakness	Acute confusional state
Hypercalcaemia	Dementia
Syndrome of inappropriate secretion of antidiuretic hormone	

Wakeful Nights

Whose problem is it? Patient, family or staff?

Causes

Physiological
Wakeful stimuli:
  light
  noise
  urinary frequency
Sleep during day:
  long siesta
  catnaps
  sedative drugs
Normal old age

Psychological
Anxiety
Depression
Fear of dying in sleep

Unrelieved symptoms
Pain
Dyspnoea
Vomiting
Incontinence
Diarrhoea
Pruritus
Restless legs

Drugs
Diuretics
Corticosteroids
Caffeine
Sympathomimetics
Hypnotic withdrawal
Alcohol (may cause
  rebound wakefulness)

Treatment Possibilities

- Explanation

- Treat primary cause
  - control disturbing symptoms
  - if night pain, consider increasing 2200 h morphine to 3 times daytime dose

- Non-drug measures
  - increase daytime activity
  - reduce light and noise at night
  - is bed comfortable?
  - hot drink at bedtime
  - soothing music
  - relaxation therapy/tape
  - discuss fears and anxieties

- Drugs
  - modify content and timing of existing drug regimen:
    corticosteroids — give as single morning dose
    anxiolytics — if receiving diazepam in daytime, convert to a single 2200 h dose
    diuretics — use fast acting loop diuretic, e.g. bumetanide, frusemide
  - prescribe a night sedative (see below)
  - prescribe a tricyclic drug if the patient is depressed or wakes early (see p. 116)
  - when all else fails, try adding chlorpromazine 50–200 mg

Choice of Night Sedative

- Temazepam 10–60 mg
  - syrup* 10 mg/5 ml — not very palatable
  - soft capsules* 10 mg, 15 mg, 20 mg and 30 mg; tablets* 10 mg, 20 mg (peak plasma concentration 0.5–1 h)
  - hard capsules* (temazepam Steinhard*) l0 mg, 20 mg (peak plasma concentration 1–1.5 h)
  - hard capsules (Restoril†) 15 mg, 30 mg (peak plasma concentration 2–3 h)—slow absorption of this formulation may reduce efficacy as a night sedative

- Triazolam tablets 0.125 mg, 0.25 mg (peak plasma concentration 0.75–2.5 h)

- Chloral derivatives
  - ☐ dichloralphenazone 650–1950 mg
  - ☐ chloral hydrate 1–2 g
- Chlormethiazole 500–1500 mg is useful in the very elderly
- Barbiturates — the authors do not use these because hepatic enzyme induction alters the metabolism of many other drugs

Weakness

Localized Weakness

May be caused by

- Peripheral nerve lesions

- Cerebral neoplasm — monoparesis, hemiparesis

- Spinal cord compression — usually bilateral (see p. 91)

Proximal muscle weakness can be caused both by cancer and by corticosteroids.

Peripheral neuropathy secondary to diabetes or vitamin B_{12} deficiency is occasionally seen in advanced cancer. Correction of hyperglycaemia or vitamin deficiency prevents further deterioration but does not result in immediate improvement. Corrective measures are therefore unnecessary in patients close to death.

Generalized Weakness

Generalized progressive weakness may mean that the patient is close to death. This should not be assumed until other causes have been considered.

Causes	Treatment possibilities
Cancer	
Progression of disease	Modify pattern of life
Anaemia	Haematinics, blood transfusion?
Hypercalcaemia	see p. 85
Hypoadrenalism	
Neuropathy	Corticosteroid
Myopathy	
Depression	Antidepressive
Treatment	
Surgery	
Chemotherapy	Guided convalescence
Radiation	
Drugs:	
diuretics	
antihypertensives	Reduce or discontinue medication
oral hypoglycaemics	
Hypokalaemia	Potassium supplements
Debility	
Insomnia	Night sedative
Exhaustion	Rest
Prolonged bedrest:	
pain	
dyspnoea	Alleviation of causal symptom
malaise	Physiotherapy
Infection	Antibiotic
Dehydration	Hydration
Malnutrition	Dietary advice (see p. 48)

Therapeutic Considerations

■ If weakness related principally to disease progression, consider a 7 day trial of corticosteroids: dexamethasone 4 mg daily *or* prednisolone 20–30 mg daily

■ Anaemia may respond to iron supplements if related to blood loss

■ Anaemia of chronic disease does not respond to the use of haematinics

■ As the patient becomes more debilitated, the benefit of blood transfusion becomes less. Treat the symptom of weakness, not the haematocrit

■ IV hyperalimentation (rarely indicated) may lead to weight gain but weakness usually persists

Hypercalcaemia

Definition

An *ionized* plasma calcium concentration above the upper limit of normal.

In most centres, the *total* plasma calcium concentration is measured. This includes both protein-bound and unbound ionized calcium. If a patient is significantly hypoalbuminaemic, the total plasma concentration may give a false impression of normality. There are several methods of 'correcting' for hypoalbuminaemia. Which one is used depends on local custom.

Generally, the following will prove satisfactory

■ In the UK, for every 1 g/L the plasma albumin concentration falls below the *mean normal albumin* for a given laboratory, add 0.02 to the total calcium concentration as measured in mmol/L

■ In the USA, for every 1 g/100 ml the plasma albumin concentration falls below 4, add 0.8 to the total calcium concentration as measured in mg/100 ml

Incidence

■ All malignant disease — 10–20%

■ Bronchus, myeloma, breast — 20–40%

Mechanisms in Cancer

Seldom associated with an occult cancer.

- **■ Metastatic**
  - □ resorption of bone induced by the metastases
  - □ prostaglandins (epithelial tumours, especially breast and renal cell)
  - □ osteoclast activating factor (myeloma, lymphoma)
  - □ vitamin D-like sterols (breast)
  - □ transient flare of hypercalcaemia may occur within 2 weeks of initiating additive hormone therapy (including tamoxifen) in breast cancer with widespread osseous metastases

■ Phosphaturic PTH-like factor in squamous cell cancer (especially bronchus, head and neck); also renal cell and bladder

This mechanism is suspected when skeletal X-ray or isotope bone scan survey fails to reveal osteolytic lesions.

Clinical Features

Severity of symptoms is not always related to degree of hypercalcaemia. Sometimes a small elevation causes definite symptoms, and vice versa.

- **■ Mild (patient ambulatory)**
  - □ fatigue
  - □ lethargy
  - □ mental dullness
  - □ weakness
  - □ anorexia
  - □ constipation

- **■ Severe (patient increasingly incapacitated)**
  - □ nausea ⎤
  - □ vomiting ⎬ → dehydration and cardiovascular collapse
  - □ ileus ⎦
  - □ confusion
  - □ drowsiness
  - □ coma

Severe symptoms may develop rapidly without a clearly defined prodrome.

Polyuria and polydipsia are not constant features.

Pain may be precipitated or exacerbated by hypercalaemia.

Diagnosis

Based on a high level of clinical suspicion.
Confirmed by appropriate blood tests.

■ Consider alternative cause, e.g. hypervitaminosis D and 'milk-alkali' syndrome

■ Check plasma chloride concentration
   □ usually < 98 mmol(mEq)/L in malignant disease
   □ usually > 103 mmol(mEq)/L in primary hyperparathyroidism

Because of impaired renal bicarbonate resorption, patients with hyperparathyroidism tend to have hyperchloraemic acidosis. Others tend to have hypochloraemic alkalosis.

■ Parathormone assay (expensive, time-consuming, can be misleading) is rarely indicated in the dying patient

Indications for Glucocorticosteroids

■ Multiple myeloma, lymphoma
   □ direct tumour suppression
   □ blocking effect of osteoclast activating factor

■ Breast, renal cell (epithelial cell tumours)
   □ antiprostaglandin effect via stabilization of cell membrane

■ Sarcoidosis, hypervitaminosis D
   □ inhibition of formation of active forms of vitamin D, thus preventing increased absorption of calcium from gastrointestinal tract

Treatment

Mild

■ Encourage high daily fluid intake (3 L) + diuresis with a loop diuretic

■ Dexamethasone 4 mg b.i.d. *or* prednisolone 20 mg b.i.d. These require several days to take effect

■ If the above ineffective, prescribe phosphate tablets 500 mg b.i.d. in place of corticosteroid. Increase by 500 mg daily every 3–7 days to a total of 3 g/day

In the UK, a 500 mg effervescent phosphate tablet is available.

In the USA, a suspension is prepared from Neutra-Phos powder; 150 ml supplies 500 mg phosphate.

Nausea and diarrhoea are the main side effects of phosphate. The latter may be a limiting factor. Beware of cumulation in renal failure. Do not use if plasma phosphate > 5 mg/dl.

Note: The above order of treatment is recommended if the primary is breast, renal cell, myeloma, lymphoma. With other cancers, we recommend the use of phosphate rather than a corticosteroid.

■ When prostaglandin production is a possible contributing factor (breast, renal cell), a NSAID should also be considered

Severe

Stop and *think*? Are you justified in correcting a potentially fatal complication in a dying patient?

Indications for urgent correction of hypercalcaemia

■ First episode or long interval since previous one

■ Previous good quality of life (in patient's opinion)

■ Patient willing to undergo IV therapy and requisite blood tests

■ Severe symptoms attributable to hypercalcaemia

■ Anticipation that corrective measures will achieve a durable effect. The results of previous treatment will serve as a guide

If urgent correction is indicated use one of the following

■ Mithramycin 25 µg/kg (approximately 1.5 mg) by IV infusion over 2 h or by slow IV injection. This is a potent inhibitor of bone resorption and lowers the plasma calcium concentration in 6–48 h

- effective in over 80% of patients
- repeat after 48 h, up to 150 μg/kg($<$10 mg) during the first week
- if renal function impaired, reduce dose to 15 μg/kg (approximately 1 mg) for a single dose; 100 μg/kg ($<$7 mg) during the first week
- do not use if bone marrow suppression or unexplained bleeding tendency

■ Pamidronate (APD)
- IV infusion 30–60 mg over 4–8 h
- give 30 mg in 500 ml of normal saline
- most respond within 3 days
- maximum effect may take 5 days
- repeat after 4–5 days if necessary
- effect often lasts 2–3 weeks
- acts by inhibiting osteoclast activity

■ Etidronate disodium
- IV infusion 7.5 mg/kg over 2–4 h = 300–600 mg in 250–500 ml of normal saline
- give daily for 3 days
- most respond within 3 days
- maximum effect may take 7 days
- acts by inhibiting osteoclast activity
- renal function must be adequate — plasma creatinine $<$180 micromol/l

Syndrome of Inappropriate Secretion of Antidiuretic Hormone

Incidence

■ All malignant disease — 1%

■ Oat-cell carcinoma of bronchus — 2%

Causes

Cancer
Oat-cell bronchus
Cerebral tumour:
  primary
  secondary
Nasopharynx
Pancreas
Colon
Prostate
Adrenal
Lymphoma
Acute myeloid
  leukaemia

Drugs
Tricyclics
Carbamazepine
Phenothiazines
Indomethacin
Chlorpropamide
Barbiturates
Opioids
Cyclophosphamide
Vincristine

Treatment
After neurosurgery

Concurrent
Meningitis
Encephalitis
Subarachnoid haemorrhage
Cerebral thrombosis
Pneumonia
Tuberculosis
Lung abscess
Trauma
Schizophrenia
Psychosis

Clinical Features

■ Plasma sodium 110–120 mmol(mEq)/L
  □ anorexia
  □ nausea
  □ vomiting
  □ lassitude
  □ confusion
  □ oedema

■ Plasma sodium < 110 mmol(mEq)/L
  □ multifocal myoclonus
  □ drowsiness
  □ fits
  □ coma

Diagnosis

■ Hyponatraemia (< 120 mmol(mEq)/L)

■ Low plasma osmolality

- Raised urine osmolality. Urine sodium concentration is
  - □ always > 20 mmol(mEq)/L
  - □ often > 50 mmol(mEq)/L

Treatment

- Mild cases — fluid restriction to 700–1000 ml/day

- If the patient finds fluid restriction unacceptable, consider demeclocycline 300 mg b.-q.i.d.
This acts by inducing a nephrogenic diabetes insipidus

- IV saline and diuretics are rarely necessary in terminal cancer

---

Spinal Cord Compression

Above Ll-L2: true cord compression
Below Ll-L2: cauda equina compression (lower motor neurone lesion)

Incidence

- All cancer patients — 5%

- ⅔ are associated with carcinoma of
  - □ breast
  - □ bronchus
  - □ prostate

- Most of the rest are associated with
  - □ hypernephroma
  - □ lymphoma
  - □ myeloma
  - □ melanoma
  - □ sarcoma
  - □ head and neck cancer

Region of Compression

- Cervical   2%

- Thoracic   80%

- Lumbar   2%
- Cervico-thoracic, thoraco-lumbar junctions   16%

Mechanism of Compression

- Metastatic spread
  - vertebral body or pedicle   85%
  - intervertebral foramina (especially lymphoma)   10%
  - intramedullary   4%
  - haematogenous (→ epidural space)   1%

Presentation

- Pain   >80%

- Weakness   >75%

- Sensory level   >50%
Note: Patient may be unaware of sensory loss until examined, especially if confined to sacrum or perineum

- Sphincter dysfunction   >40%

Pain

The following may or may not be present

- Local bone pain

- Root compression pain

- Cord compression pain (cuff or garter pain, often around thighs, knees or calves)

Diagnosis

- History

- Clinical findings

- X-ray shows vertebral metastasis/collapse at appropriate level in 80%

- Bone scan does not often yield additional information

- Myelogram if in doubt and if necessary for planning treatment

- CT (computed tomography) avoids the discomfort of a myelogram but may be negative even with complete block. CT can be used if patient refuses myelogram

- Magnetic resonance imaging is the investigation of choice but is not yet widely available

Therapeutic Guidelines

- Dexamethasone
  - ☐ 12 mg PO stat
    6 mg q.i.d. thereafter ⎫
  - ☐ 100 mg IV stat   ⎬ Alternative regimens
    24 mg PO q.i.d. for 3 days
    rapid reduction to 4 mg q.i.d. ⎭

- Radiation therapy concurrently

- Decompressive laminectomy. Consider if
  - ☐ symptoms and signs (other than pain) progress relentlessly despite radiation and high dose dexamethasone regimen
  - ☐ relapse after maximum radiation given
  - ☐ solitary vertebral metastasis
  - ☐ diagnosis in doubt

Patients with an incomplete block fare best
Recovery more likely after partial lesions of cauda equina
Loss of sphincter function is a bad prognostic sign

Acute Confusional State

Definition

Confusion is the result of 'mental clouding'. This leads to a disturbance of comprehension and poor concentration.

Synonym — Acute organic brain syndrome

Clinical Features

- Poor concentration

- Impairment of short-term memory

- Disorientation

- Misperceptions
- Paranoid delusions
- Hallucinations
- Rambling incoherent speech
- Restlessness
- Noisy/aggressive behaviour

There may be associated drowsiness. Psychomotor activity may be increased or decreased.

Increased activity may be associated with overactivity of the autonomic nervous system — facial flushing, dilated pupils, injected conjunctivae, tachycardia, sweating.

Confusion about Confusion

Patients manifesting the following are sometimes wrongly said to be confused

- Not taking in what is said
  - deaf
  - anxious
  - too ill to concentrate
- Forgetful
- Disorientation
  - time   } does not warrant the label 'confusion'
  - place   } if sole abnormality
- Misperception
- Muddled speech
  - poor concentration
  - nominal dysphasia
- Hallucination

It is important to distinguish between pathological hallucinations and

- Hypnogogic hallucinations
- Hypnopompic hallucinations
- Vivid nightmares

Hypnogogic and hypnopompic hallucinations are normal though more common in patients receiving drugs with sedative effects. A hypnopompic hallucination is a hallucinatory extension of a dream into wakefulness. In contrast, hypnogogic hallucinations occur as a person is dropping off to sleep. If these common, normal phenomena are called 'hallucinations' without explanation, this will cause anxiety because of the common assumption that hallucinations means one is going mad.

Although unpleasant, the content of a patient's nightmares may reflect fears about death that the patient has not yet been able to face up to at a conscious level.

Causes of Confusion

Cancer:
  systemic effect
  cerebral involvement
	Drugs:
	  sedative
	  stimulant
	  antiParkinsonian
	  cimetidine
	  digoxin

Infection	
Dehydration	Vitamin deficiency

Unfamiliar excessive stimuli:
  too hot
  too cold
  wet bed
  crumbs in bed
  creases in sheets
  pain and fatigue
  constipation
  retention of urine
  pruritus
	Alcohol deprivation
	
	Drug withdrawal
	
	Biochemical derangement:
	  hypercalcaemia
	  hyponatraemia
	  hypoglycaemia
	  hyperglycaemia

Change of environment
 	
Anxiety
	Cerebral anoxia:
	  anaemia
	  cardiac failure
	  hypoxia

Depression	Organ failure:
	  hepatic
	  renal

Treatment

Explanation

- Stress that patient is not going mad
- Stress that often there are lucid intervals
- Continue to treat the patient with courtesy and respect

Note: Hallucinations, nightmares and misperceptions tend to reflect the patient's unresolved fears and anxieties.

General measures

- Restraints should not be used
- Bed rails should be avoided — they can be dangerous
- Patient should be allowed to walk about accompanied
- Allay fear and suspicion, and reduce misperceptions by
  □ using a night light
  □ not changing the position of the patient's bed
  □ explaining every procedure and event in detail
  □ the presence of a family member or close friend

Drugs

Use drugs only if symptoms are marked, persistent and cause distress to patient and/or family.

Review after several hours if a sedative drug is prescribed, as symptoms may be exacerbated.

Consider the following measures

- Reduction in medication

- Oxygen if cyanosed

- Dexamethasone (4 mg t.-q.i.d.) if cerebral tumour

- Diazepam 5–10 mg PO or PR if agitated

- Haloperidol 1.5–15 mg PO or IM if
  □ hallucinated
  □ paranoid
  □ diazepam fails to relieve

Initial dose of diazepam *or* haloperidol depends on previous medication, weight, age and severity of symptoms. Subsequent doses depend on initial response (see pp. 109 and 113).

Daily or b.i.d. maintenance doses usually adequate; sometimes more frequent administration is necessary.

The following are useful alternative preparations

■ Chlormethiazole*
  □ in very elderly
  □ if alcohol withdrawal suspected

■ Chlorpromazine if haloperidol fails and the therapeutic aim is to induce somnolence

■ Midazolam for continuous SC use (see p. 114)

Dementia

Definition

A syndrome of cognitive (intellectual) impairment, in which one or more of the brain's higher integrative functions is affected; namely, perception, memory, calculation, capacity for judgement, use of language.

Synonym — Chronic organic brain syndrome

Clinical Features

■ Dementia is not usually associated with an impaired level of consciousness

■ Typically, dementia develops slowly but confusion rapidly

■ Some patients with cancer appear to develop dementia rapidly — this may cause difficulty in diagnosis

Comparison between organic brain syndromes

Confusion		*Dementia*
Mental clouding		Brain damage
(information not taken in)		(information not retained)

+	Poor concentration	+
+	Impaired short-term memory	+
+	Disorientation	+
+	Living in the past	+
+	Misinterpretations	+
+ +	Hallucinations	–
+	Psychosis	–

Speech rambling and incoherent	Stereotyped and limited
Variable	Constant
Often aware and anxious	Often unaware and unconcerned

Causes

Most patients with dementia have the idiopathic form
(Alzheimer's disease). In others it is secondary to cerebral
atherosclerosis/cerebral thrombosis.

Dementia may be precipitated or exacerbated by many factors.
Debility, depression, drug intoxication or a confusional state may
unmask a previously well compensated dementia or exacerbate
one of moderate degree.

Some patients manifest symptoms and signs of both dementia
and confusion. The concurrence of cognitive impairment and
mental clouding can cause major management problems.

■ Some patients with dementia develop cancer

■ Some patients with cancer develop dementia

Therapeutic Guidelines

■ Explanation to the patient if possible, and to the family

■ Correct reversible causal factors. Even in a dying patient the physician needs to be reasonably certain that reversible causes of dementia are not overlooked

---

Potentially treatable exacerbating factors in dementia

Psychiatric disorders
Depression (pseudodementia)
Confusional states

Infection
Systemic
Intracranial:
  cytomegalic virus
  fungal meningitis
  tuberculous meningitis
  neurosyphilis

Intractable tumours
Subdural haematoma
Meningioma
Glioma
Metastases

Hydrocephalus

Metabolic disorders
Organ failure
Hepatic encephalopathy

Endocrine disorders
Myxoedema
Hyperthyroidism
Hypoparathyroidism
Hypopituitarism

Deficiency states
Thiamine
Nicotinic acid
Hydroxycobalamin
Folic acid

Drugs
Alcohol
Anticonvulsants
Barbiturates
Belladonna alkaloids
Benzodiazepines
Bromides
Cimetidine
Disulfiram
Lithium
Methyldopa
Neuroleptics
Opioids
Tricyclics

Miscellaneous
Connective tissue disorders
Sarcoidosis
Haemodialysis

Metallic toxins
Arsenic
Lead
Manganese
Mercury

Volatile agents
Alcohols, etc
Carbon disulphide
Carbon monoxide
Hydrocarbons
Organic solvents

---

5 PSYCHOTROPIC DRUGS

Classification
Anticholinergic effects
Extrapyramidal drug
    reactions
Phenothiazines

Haloperidol
Benzodiazepines
Diazepam
Midazolam
Antidepressives

Classification

Neuroleptics

- □ phenothiazines
- □ butyrophenones
- □ thioxanthenes
- □ benzamides

Anxiolytic sedatives

- □ meprobamate
- □ barbiturates
- □ benzodiazepines
- □ hydroxyzine
- □ buspirone

Antidepressives

- □ tricyclic and related drugs
- □ MAOI
- □ other

Psychostimulants

- □ caffeine
- □ amphetamine
- □ methylphenidate
- □ cocaine

Psychodysleptics (hallucinogens)

- □ cannabis
- □ lysergic acid diethylamide (LSD)
- □ mescaline
- □ psilocybin
- □ dimethyltryptophan (DMT)

A few patients respond paradoxically when prescribed, e.g. diazepam (become more distressed) or amitriptyline (become wakeful and restless at night).

Other patients will derive little benefit from a benzodiazepine, e.g. diazepam but will be helped by a neuroleptic, e.g. haloperidol.

As a general rule, smaller doses should be used in patients with advanced cancer than with more robust patients, especially if already receiving morphine or another psychotropic drug.

After an initial small test dose, the dose can be increased fairly quickly (e.g. every 2–3 days) until troublesome unwanted effects appear or until a satisfactory response is obtained

There may be a need for a subsequent *reduction* in dose because of drug cumulation. As with analgesics, close supervision is essential particularly during the first few days.

Anticholinergic Effects

> 'dry as a bone,
> blind as a bat,
> red as a beet,
> hot as a hare,
> mad as a hatter'

- ■ Dry mouth

- ■ Blurred vision (mydriasis and loss of accommodation)

- ■ Palpitations
  Extrasystoles
  Arrhythmias

Also related to noradrenaline potentiation and a quinidine-like action

- ■ Heartburn (reduced tone in lower oesophageal sphincter)

- Constipation

- Hesitancy of micturition
  Retention of urine

Causes

Belladonna alkaloids	Antihistamines
	chlorpheniramine
Neuroleptics	cyclizine
phenothiazines	meclozine†
haloperidol	hydroxyzine
Antidepressives	Antispasmodics
tricyclics	propantheline
mianserin*	oxybutynin
	mebeverine

Extrapyramidal Drug Reactions

Extrapyramidal reactions are caused by

- Neuroleptic drugs
  □ phenothiazines
  □ haloperidol

- Metoclopramide

Parkinsonism

Parkinsonism develops at any stage after commencement of treatment, although not usually before the second week. It is most common in the over 60s.

- Intention tremor

- Muscle rigidity

- Poverty of facial expression

- Sialorrhoea (drooling)

- Shuffling gait

Treatment

Use an anticholinergic antiParkinsonian drug

- Benztropine 1–2 mg IV/IM → 2 mg PO daily-b.i.d. *or*
- Procyclidine 5–10 mg IV/IM → 2.5–5 mg PO t.i.d.

Akathisia

Akathisia is a form of motor restlessness in which the subject is compelled to pace up and down or to change the body position frequently. It is seen in Parkinson's disease and in association with neuroleptic drugs, usually in high doses.

It may develop as early as the second week of treatment. If the drug is continued, it may progress to Parkinsonism. It is most common in the 16–60 age range.

- Compulsive floor pacing
- Body rocking when standing
- Weight shifting from foot to foot
- Patients feel and look anxious

Treatment

- Consider reducing causal drug
- Prescribe anticholinergic antiParkinsonian drug b.-t.i.d.
- If response only partial, add diazepam
- In resistant cases, discontinue causal drug

Acute Dystonias

Acute dystonias develop abruptly within days of starting treatment, and are accompanied by anxiety. They are most common in young, female patients.

- Trismus
- Torticollis
- Facial spasm
- Oculogyric crisis
- Opisthotonos

Treatment

- Benztropine 1–2 mg *or* procyclidine 5–10 mg IV/IM for immediate relief. If necessary, repeat after 30 min

- Continue treatment with a standard oral anticholinergic antiParkinsonian drug (see above)

- Consider discontinuing or reducing dose of causal drug

- If caused by metoclopramide, substitute domperidone*

Tardive Dyskinesia

Tardive ('late') dyskinesia is caused by the long-term administration of drugs that block dopamine receptors, particularly D_2 receptors. It is caused most often by potent neuroleptic drugs and also by metoclopramide.

Tardive dyskinesia occurs in 20% of patients receiving a neuroleptic for more than 3 months. Women, the elderly and those on high doses (e.g. chlorpromazine 300 mg/day) are most commonly affected.

In younger patients, tardive dyskinesia may occur if neuroleptic treatment is stopped abruptly, but not if tailed off gradually.

Typically, tardive dyskinesia manifests as involuntary stereotyped chewing movements of the tongue and orofacial muscles.

In younger patients, tardive dyskinesia may present as abnormal posturing of the limbs and tonic contractions of the neck and trunk muscles causing torticollis, lordosis or scoliosis.

The involuntary movements are made worse by anxiety and reduced by drowsiness and in sleep.

Tardive dyskinesia seldom causes subjective distress, unless associated with akathisia — this is seen in 25% of cases.

Early diagnosis

'Open your mouth and stick out your tongue'
The following indicate a developing tardive dyskinesia

- Worm-like movements of the tongue

- Inability to protrude tongue for more than a few seconds

Treatment

■ Withdrawal of causal agent leads to resolution in 30% in 3 months and a further 40% in 5 years. Sometimes irreversible particularly in the elderly

■ Often responds poorly to drug therapy; anticholinergic antiParkinsonian drugs may exacerbate

■ Tetrabenazine — depletes presynaptic biogenic amine stores and blocks postsynaptic dopamine receptors. Best not used in depressed patients. Increase dose slowly to avoid troublesome hypotension. Start with 12.5 mg t.i.d. → 25 mg t.i.d.

■ Reserpine — depletes presynaptic biogenic amine stores. May be used in place of tetrabenazine; causes similar unwanted effects

■ Levodopa — may produce long-term benefit after causing initial deterioration

■ GABA antagonists — baclofen, sodium valproate, diazepam and clonazepam have all been tried with inconsistent results

■ Increasing the dose of the causal drug — paradoxically, this may help but should be considered only in desperation

Phenothiazines

Classification

Ethylamino derivatives
□ promethazine

Propylamino derivatives

□ chlorpromazine
□ methotrimeprazine
□ promazine
□ trimeprazine

Piperazine derivatives (halogenation of Rl side chain)

□ fluphenazine
□ perphenazine
□ prochlorperazine

☐ thiethylperazine
☐ trifluoperazine

Piperidine derivatives

☐ ethopropazine
☐ thioridazine

Properties and Uses

■ Antiemetic — particularly piperazine derivatives

■ Antipsychotic

■ Anxiolytic

■ Night sedative

■ Rectal tenesmoid pain

} particularly propylamino derivatives

■ Analgesic — only methotrimeprazine

The sedative and hypotensive effects of methotrimeprazine limit its usefulness. Although prescribed at some centres, methotrimeprazine is not used by the authors.

Limitations

■ Anticholinergic effects — particularly piperidines

■ Drowsiness

■ Postural hypotension

■ Extrapyramidal reactions — particularly piperazines

General Comments

■ Except when used as a night sedative, need to be given t.i.d. or more often

■ Useful as an anxiolytic for patients who react paradoxically to diazepam

■ Piperidine derivatives have little or no place in terminal care. Thioridazine has no antiemetic effect and a high incidence of anticholinergic effects

- Generally, parenteral administration should be IM because too irritant SC

- Prochlorperazine may be given by intermittent SC injection but if it causes erythema or discomfort, given IM

Therapeutic Guidelines

Phenothiazines are manufactured in syrup, tablet, suppository and parenteral forms. Specific availability varies from country to country.

- Antiemetic
  - fluphenazine (Moditen*, Prolixin†) 1–2 mg b.i.d.
  - prochlorperazine 5–10 mg q4–8h
  - perphenazine 2–4 mg q6–8h
  - trifluoperazine 1–2 mg b.i.d.

- Antipsychotic
  - chlorpromazine 10–100 mg q4–8h
  - trifluoperazine 5 mg b.-q.i.d.

- Anxiolytic
  - prochlorperazine 5–10 mg q4–8h
  - chlorpromazine 10–100 mg q4–8h
  - trifluoperazine 5 mg b.-q.i.d.

- Night sedative
  - chlorpromazine 25–200 mg nocte
  - methotrimeprazine 25–100 mg nocte

- Rectal tenesmoid analgesic
  - chlorpromazine 10–25 mg q8h

Haloperidol

Properties and Uses

- Antiemetic

- Antipsychotic

- Anxiolytic

Limitations

- Anticholinergic effects
- Extrapyramidal reactions
- Drowsiness

General Comments

- Plasma half-life = 16 h; can usually be given once daily
- In higher doses (⩾ 5 mg) has a distinct sedative effect, and may substitute satisfactorily for a night sedative
- Extrapyramidal effects more likely at daily doses of ⩾ 5 mg As these do not occur consistently, it is better *not* to administer an antiParkinsonian drug prophylactically but to treat if symptoms develop
- Anxiolytic of choice for patients with paranoid or psychotic traits
- Haloperidol compared with chlorpromazine
  - □ *more* antiemetic
    extrapyramidal reactions
  - □ *less* sedation
    anticholinergic effects
    cardiovascular effects

Therapeutic Guidelines

Haloperidol is available in solution, capsule* (0.5 mg), tablet (1†, 1.5*, 2†, 5, 10 mg) and parenteral forms.

- Antiemetic (for chemical/toxic causes of vomiting)
  - □ 1–1.5 mg stat and nocte (= standard dose for morphine-induced vomiting)
  - □ 3–5 mg nocte if smaller dose not effective
  - □ 5–20 mg nocte, or in divided dosage, for chemotherapy related vomiting and in patients with biochemically determined vomiting (e.g. hypercalcaemia and uraemia)
- Antipsychotic
  - □ 1.5–3 mg stat and nocte in the elderly (70+)
  - □ 5 mg stat and nocte in the younger patient or if poor response in elderly

□ 10–20 mg nocte, or in divided dosage, if poor response
- Anxiolytic
  □ 5 mg stat and nocte
  □ 10–20 mg nocte, or in divided dosage, if poor response

Benzodiazepines

A group of anxiolytic sedative drugs.

Despite a non-linear relationship, the plasma half-life of a benzodiazepine and its pharmacologically active metabolites reflects the duration of its effects.

Those with long half-lives can be used as 'once a day' anxiolytics, tend to cumulate when given repeatedly, and are more likely to cause drowsiness and impairment of psychomotor skills.

Classification

Half-life here refers to the plasma half-life of the named drug and its pharmacologically active metabolites.

- Short acting (half-life <5 h)
  □ midazolam
  □ triazolam

- intermediate acting (half-life 5–25 h)
  □ temazepam
  □ oxazepam
  □ lorazepam
  □ flunitrazepam

- Long acting (half-life >25 h)
  □ chlordiazepoxide
  □ clonazepam
  □ chlorazepate
  □ diazepam
  □ flurazepam
  □ nitrazepam

Clinical Indications

- Insomnia

- Anxiety

- Muscle tension/spasm

- Multifocal myoclonus

- Fits

Routes of Administration

- The oral route is best when used as a night sedative, anxiolytic or muscle relaxant

- Diazepam is available as both a suppository and a rectal solution* (Stesolid)

- Parenteral diazepam is an oil-based preparation and should *not* be given IM as absorption is slow and variable. IV diazepam may cause thrombophlebitis

- Midazolam and flunitrazepam are water-soluble and can be given SC, IM and IV

- IV lorazepam is less likely than diazepam to cause thrombophlebitis and respiratory depression but causes more amnesia. As it exhibits a variable delay between administration and onset of action, it is *not* recommended

Therapeutic Guidelines

- Night sedative
  - □ short acting drugs (see p. 82)

- Anxiolytic
  - □ long acting drugs:
       diazepam 2–20 mg nocte, occasionally b.-t.i.d.
  - □ intermediate acting drugs:
       lorazepam 1–2 mg b.-t.i.d.
       temazepam *hard* capsules (Restoril†) 10 mg b.-t.i.d.

- Muscle relaxant
  - □ diazepam 2–20 mg nocte
Baclofen (*not* a benzodiazepine) is a useful alternative, particularly if anxiety is not an associated problem and if diazepam too sedative.

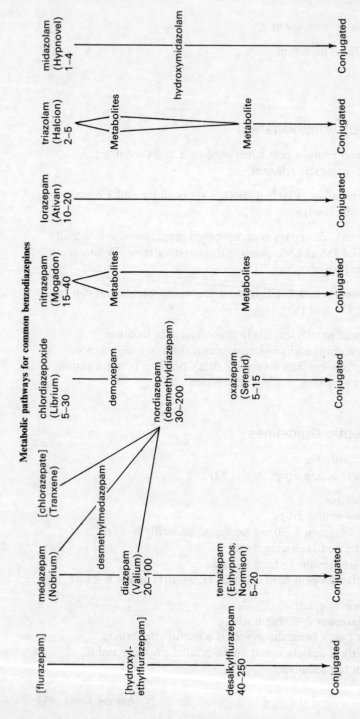

Metabolic pathways for common benzodiazepines

midazolam (Hypnovel) 1–4	→ hydroxymidazolam → Conjugated

Note: 1. Names in square brackets = pro-drugs or drug precursors that do not reach systemic circulation as such in clinically important amounts.
2. Figures refer to plasma elimination half-lives.
3. Lorazepam does not use the P450 hepatic metabolic pathway and avoids drug interactions dependent upon competition for this pathway.

- Anticonvulsant
  - □ diazepam
  - □ midazolam
  - □ clonazepam

Clonazepam is very potent and would need to be introduced in very small doses in patients with advanced cancer, e.g. 0.5 mg nocte, rising by 0.5 mg every 3–5 days up to 2–4 mg, occasionally more.

Diazepam

Properties and Uses

- Anxiolytic
- Night sedative
- Muscle relaxant
- Anticonvulsant

Diazepam may be used as an antiemetic adjuvant for cisplatin-induced vomiting. It is not anticholinergic.

Limitations

- Daytime drowsiness
- Muscular flaccidity
- Postural hypotension

General Comments

- Plasma half-life = 2 days; can usually be given once a day *at bedtime*

- Patients occasionally react paradoxically, i.e. become more distressed; if so change to haloperidol *or* chlorpromazine

- If drowsiness develops because of cumulation, reduce the dose

- If patient does not sleep at night, daytime drowsiness more likely

- Diazepam acts faster PO or PR than IM as preparation is oil-based

- IV may cause thrombophlebitis; inject slowly and dilute with blood. An oil-in-water emulsion (Diazemuls*) should be used if available

Therapeutic Guidelines

- Initial dose depends on patient's previous experience of diazepam and related drugs, intensity of distress and urgency of relief:
  - □ 2 mg — useful and safe in the elderly (70 +)
  - □ 5 mg — standard initial dose
  - □ 10 mg — for severe distress, especially in younger patients

- Repeat hourly until the desired effect is achieved, and then decide on appropriate maintenance regimen

- Rectal diazepam is a useful alternative in a crisis or if moribund
  - □ suppositories 10 mg
  - □ rectal solution* (Stesolid) 5–10 mg in 2.5 ml
  - □ parenteral formulation via a cannula

Patterns of Use

- 'As required' — best initial way in elderly, and for acute (possibly transient) episodes of anxiety

- Regularly at bedtime — best for those with prolonged anxiety. Also is used for muscle spasm or general stiffness

- More than daily (e.g. 1000/1400, 2200 h or 1000, 1800, 2200 h) in bedfast patients with intractable terminal agitation Aim = a reduction in the number of hours the patient is awake and distressed. Occasionally, it is necessary to keep a patient asleep because he is overwhelmingly distressed when awake.

Midazolam

Properties and Uses

- Anaesthetic induction agent

- Sedative for minor procedures

- Sedative for terminal agitation

- Anticonvulsant

Midazolam v diazepam

■ Sedation — midazolam is twice as potent

■ Anticonvulsant — midazolam is equipotent

■ Midazolam is water-soluble and can be given SC, IM and IV

Sedation for minor procedures (10 mg/5 ml)

■ Doses varies mainly according to age

■ Usually between 2–10 mg

■ In elderly, give 1 mg and then 0.5 mg/min until sedated

Sedation for terminal agitation (10 mg/2 ml)

■ SC/IM 5 mg stat → SC infusion 30 mg/24 h

■ 5 mg SC/IM every hour if not settled; increase to 40 mg/24 h if two 'as required' doses needed after starting SC infusion

■ If failed on diazepam 20 mg PO/PR, consider 20 mg midazolam SC/IM stat → SC infusion 60 mg/24 h and 10–20 mg SC/IM every hour if not settled

■ Occasionally a patient needs 100 mg in 20 ml/24 h

Sedation for catastrophic emergencies (10 mg/5 ml; 10 mg/2 ml)

■ Acute tracheal compression (→ acute asphyxia) and massive tracheobronchial haemorrhage are *rare*

■ If not immediately fatal, the distressed patient may benefit by being rendered unconscious with IV midazolam 5–20 mg

Anticonvulsant (10 mg/2ml)

■ IM/IV 10 mg stat → SC infusion 30 mg/24 h

■ 10 mg SC/IM every hour if still fitting; increase to 60 mg/24 h if two 'as required' doses needed after starting SC infusion

Antidepressives

Classification

Tricyclic drugs

- [ ] amitriptyline
- [ ] clomipramine
- [ ] desipramine
- [ ] dothiepin*

Related drugs

- [ ] mianserin*
- [ ] iprindole*
- [ ] maprotiline

MAOI

- [ ] phenelzine
- [ ] isocarboxazid
- [ ] tranylcypromine

Other

- [ ] flupenthixol*
- [ ] fluvoxamine*
- [ ] tryptophan
- [ ] lithium

Lithium is used increasingly to prevent recurrent depression both unipolar and bipolar (manic-depressive); also used in combination with tryptophan and a tricyclic drug *or* MAOI in unresponsive depression.

The term 'tricyclic antidepressive' is outmoded because

■ There are now 1-, 2- and 4- ring drugs with similar properties

■ Depression is only one of several indications for their use in cancer

Tricyclic and related antidepressives are the drugs of choice in the treatment of depression. In severe drug-resistant cases, electroconvulsive therapy (ECT) may be necessary.

These drugs are preferred to MAOI because they are more

effective antidepressives and do not cause the dangerous interactions with certain foods and drugs.

Interactions with MAOI

Tyramine-containing foods	Biogenic monoamine enhancing drugs
Cheese	Sympathomimetics
Pickled herring	Levodopa
Broad bean pods	Tetrabenazine
Meat or yeast extracts:	Reserpine
Bovril	Other antidepressives
Oxo	
Marmite	
Alcohol	

The concurrent use of a MAOI and pethidine/meperidine may lead to respiratory depression, restlessness, hypotension, and possibly coma. This is possibly related to the inhibition of the hepatic demethylation of pethidine.

Pharmacology

Tricyclic and related drugs have a range of actions

- Blockade of reuptake by presynaptic terminals of
  - serotonin (5-hydroxytryptamine, 5HT)
  - noradrenaline (norepinephrine)

- Receptor blockade
  - muscarinic cholinergic
  - H_1-histaminergic
  - α_1-adrenergic

A synopsis of some of these effects is given in the table (see p. 118)

- Sedation is related to blockade of the central H_1-histaminergic receptors

- Hypotension is related to blockade of the α_1-adrenergic receptors

- H_1-histaminergic and α_1-adrenergic potency are closely correlated

Pharmacological properties of some antidepressive drugs

Antidepressive drugs	Type	Plasma elimination half-life (h)	Noradrenaline uptake inhibition	Serotonin uptake inhibition	Anticholinergic effects	Sedative effects
Tricyclic compounds:						
imipramine[1]	tertiary amine	4–18	++	++	+++	++
amitriptyline[2]	tertiary amine	10–25	+	+++	+++	+++
clomipramine	tertiary amine	16–20	+	+++	++	++
nortriptyline	secondary amine	13–93	+++	+	++	0
desipramine	secondary amine	12–61	+++	0	+	0
protriptyline	secondary amine	54–198	+++	+	+++	0
doxepin[3]	tertiary amine	8–25	+	+	++	++
dothiepin*	tertiary amine	14–40	+	+	+	++
Related compounds:						
viloxazine* (bicyclic)	secondary amine	2–5	+++	0	0	0
maprotiline (bridged tricyclic)	secondary amine	27–58	+++	+	+	+
mianserin*[4]	tertiary amine	8–19	0	0	0	++
Unrelated compounds:						
trazodone[4]		4	0	+	0	++

1 Metabolized to desipramine.
2 Metabolized to nortriptyline.
3 Metabolized to desmethyldodoxepin (β half-life 33–81 h).
4 Inhibits presynaptic α_2 receptors.
Pharmacological activity: 0 = none; + = slight; ++ = moderate; +++ = marked.

From Ashton CH 1989 *Brain Systems, Disorders and Psychotropic Drugs*. Oxford Medical Publications, Oxford

- There is no correlation between anticholinergic potency and sedation
  - □ protriptyline is non-sedative but moderately anticholinergic
  - □ mianserin* is moderately sedative but is not anticholinergic
- Sedative effects tend to be more common in physically ill patients, particularly if receiving other psychoactive drugs, including morphine
- The antidepressive effect of the tricyclic drugs is related to the enhancement of the actions of the monoamines — noradrenaline and serotonin

Tricyclics and Pain

- The results of controlled trials of tricyclic drugs for deafferentation pain are not entirely consistent
- Partial relief of deafferentation pain is sometimes seen as early as 3 days after beginning treatment in contrast to 5–14 for an antidepressive effect
- Drugs that preferentially block serotonin reuptake (e.g. amitriptyline, clomipramine, imipramine) are probably more effective at relieving deafferentation pain than drugs that preferentially block noradrenaline reuptake (e.g. nortriptyline, desipramine)
- Both serotonergic and noradrenergic neurones in the brainstem project to and inhibit nociceptive cells in the spinal cord
- Tricyclic drugs administered systemically or intrathecally enhance the analgesic effect of morphine given systemically
- Pain relief with tricyclic drugs is independent of an antidepressive effect
- The mechanisms by which tricyclic drugs relieve depression and pain may be different

Uses of Tricyclic and Related Drugs

- Depression
- Early morning insomnia
- Deafferentation pain

- Urgency of micturition
- Urge incontinence
- Nocturnal enuresis
- Bladder spasms

Choice of Drug

This will depend on the intended use. The table on p. 118 provides a rational basis for prescribing.

Four or five drugs suffice to cover all necessary options

- Desipramine (non-sedative, minimal anticholinergic effects)
- Dothiepin* or mianserin* (sedative, minimal or no anticholinergic effects)
- Amitriptyline (marked serotonin reuptake inhibition, marked anticholinergic effects)
- Clomipramine (marked serotonin reuptake inhibition, moderate anticholinergic effects)
- Nortriptyline (non-sedative)

Depressed cancer patients are often also anxious and best results may be obtained with a sedative drug, e.g. dothiepin* or mianserin*.

Clomipramine is the tricyclic of choice for patients with depression associated with obsessional features.

A sedative antidepressive is required to correct early morning insomnia.

For deafferentation pain, amitriptyline clomipramine *or* imipramine are good choices.

For bladder spasms and urgency caused by detrusor hyperreflexia, amitriptyline is the drug of choice.

Therapeutic Considerations

In practice, all tricyclic drugs can be given in a single dose at bedtime.

- If patient experiences early morning drowsiness, or takes a long time settling at night, advise to take 1–2 h before bedtime

■ Anticholinergic cardiac effects are occasionally troublesome, but a cardiac history is not a contraindication to careful use

■ A small number of patients are stimulated by amitriptyline and experience insomnia, unpleasant vivid dreams, myoclonus and physical restlessness. In these patients, administer amitriptyline in the morning or change to mianserin*

■ Mianserin* acts *presynaptically* by blocking α_2 adrenergic receptors. This results in increased noradrenaline release and turnover. Mianserin* is about 2.5 times more potent than amitriptyline, i.e. mianserin* 60 mg = amitriptyline 150 mg

■ Mianserin* has occasionally been associated with agranulocytosis. This is generally reversible on stopping treatment. Most cases have occurred in the first month of treatment; the manufacturers recommend monthly blood counts for the first 3 months. Agranulocytosis is more common in the elderly and in patients with organic disease

■ When an antidepressive is used to treat deafferentation pain, benefit may be seen as early as 3–5 days

■ An antidepressive effect may also be seen as soon as this, though it commonly takes longer

■ Relatively small doses are often efficacious in relieving depression in debilitated cancer patients

■ It is wise to commence with a small dose of a tricyclic in patients with advanced cancer, particulary if frail or over 70

Dose	Elderly frail/ outpatient	Younger patient/ inpatient
25 mg nocte	Week 1	Day 1
50 mg nocte	Week 2	Day 2–4
75 mg nocte	Week 3 + 4	Day 5–21
100 mg nocte	Week 5 + 6	Week 3 + 4
150 mg nocte	Week 7 + 8	Week 5 + 6

6 RESPIRATORY SYMPTOMS

Cough   'Death rattle'
Dyspnoea   Hyoscine
Hiccup

Cough

Definition

A complex respiratory reflex designed to expel foreign particulate
matter and excess mucus from the trachea and main bronchi.

Incidence

All terminal cancer — 50%
Bronchogenic cancer — 80%

Relevant Physiology

Each cough comprises a three phase mechanism which produces a
high velocity expiratory airflow. A shearing force is created which
aids the expulsion of mucus and foreign materials.

■ Inspiratory phase (glottis open)

■ Compressive phase (glottis closed) → increased intrathoracic
pressure

■ Expiratory phase (glottis open) → explosive release of
trapped air

The inspiratory and expiratory phases are mediated primarily by
thoracic and abdominal muscles. Both will be adversely affected
by thoracic and abdominal pain, weakness and depressed
consciousness.

A closed glottis is not an essential part of the compressive phase.
The expiratory muscles are capable of producing elevated
intrathoracic pressures with an open glottis.

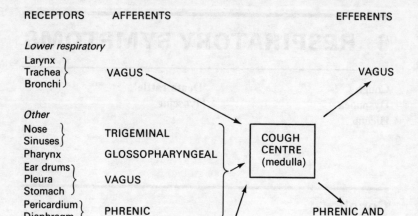

RECEPTORS	AFFERENTS	EFFERENTS

Lower respiratory
Larynx ⎫
Trachea ⎬ VAGUS
Bronchi ⎭

Other
Nose ⎫
Sinuses ⎭ TRIGEMINAL
Pharynx   GLOSSOPHARYNGEAL
Ear drums ⎫
Pleura ⎬ VAGUS
Stomach ⎭
Pericardium ⎫
Diaphragm ⎭ PHRENIC

CEREBRAL CORTEX

COUGH CENTRE (medulla)

VAGUS

PHRENIC AND SPINAL MOTOR NERVES

Causes

Cancer	*Debility*
Mechanical irritation of:	Chest infection
pharynx	
trachea	*Concurrent*
bronchial tree	Postnasal drip
pleura	Cigarettes
pericardium	Chronic obstructive pulmonary
diaphragm	disease (COPD)
	Asthma
Treatment	Heart failure
Radiation-induced fibrosis	

Types of Cough

- Wet + patient able to cough effectively (productive)

- Wet + patient too weak to cough effectively (non-productive)

- Dry (non-productive)

Treatment Possibilities

- Explanation

- Treat concurrent causes
  - postnasal drip — antihistamine
  - bronchospasm — bronchodilator
  - heart failure — diuretic
  - infection — antibiotic
  - cigarettes — stop smoking

Note: It takes 2–4 weeks to obtain significant antitussive benefit from stopping smoking. Will the patient live this long?

- Modification of pathological process
  - radiation therapy
  - chemotherapy
  - corticosteroids

- Non-drug measures
  - advise how to cough effectively (it is impossible to cough¨ effectively lying on your back)
  - postural drainage
  - physiotherapy

- Mucolytics ('expectorants')

A mucolytic aids expectoration by making bronchial secretions less viscid. It does not stimulate the cough reflex directly.
  - water:
      humidification
      saline 2–5% in nebulizer
      steam inhalations
  - chemical inhalations:
      compound benzoin tincture (Friar's balsam)
      carbol
      menthol and eucalyptus*
  - irritant mucolytics:
      ammonium chloride
      guaiphenesin (Robitussin)
      ipecacuanha
      potassium iodide† (SSKI)
      terpin hydrate
    mechanisms of action obscure. Said to stimulate the production of more profuse, less viscid bronchial secretions. Also gastric irritants and may cause nausea and vomiting

☐ chemical mucolytics:
    tyloxapol* (Alevaire)
    acetylcisteine† (Mucomist)
best given as a nebulized solution. They modify the chemical structure of sputum and reduce its viscosity. Evidence of efficacy is limited. Their use should be discouraged

■ Antitussives
Peripheral
☐ pharynx:
    simple linctus
☐ lung:
    benzonatate† (Tessalon perls) — inhibits stretch receptor reflex
    nebulized bupivacaine — blocks cough receptors:
        mechanical (carina)
        chemical (bronchioles)
Central
☐ non-opioids:
    isoaminile*
☐ opioid derivatives:
    dextromethorphan
    levopropoxyphene† (Novrad)
    pholcodine
☐ opioid:
    codeine
    dihydrocodeine*
    hydrocodone† (Hycodan)
    morphine
    methadone
    hydromorphone†

Pethidine/meperidine is not antitussive.

Most commercial cough preparations contain subtherapeutic doses of an antitussive, a mucolytic, a sympathomimetic and an antihistamine, in a demulcent (soothing) vehicle. The vehicle is probably the most important component and, like simple syrup, acts by reducing pharyngeal sensitivity.

Therapeutic Guidelines

Treatment depends on both the cause and the therapeutic goal. In the dying patient the goal is comfort.

Wet cough + patient able to cough effectively

■ Humidification of inspired air
  □ room humidifier
  □ steam inhalations

■ Education on how to cough more effectively

■ Postural drainage and percussion

■ Antibiotic?

■ Bronchodilator?

■ Mucolytic

Wet cough + patient too weak to cough effectively

■ Antitussive
  □ simple linctus 10 ml q2–4h
  □ codeine 30–60 mg q4h *or*
    morphine 5–20 mg q4h
  □ benzonatate† 100 mg q4–6h
Different types of antitussives may be used in combination
because of different modes of action. It is nonsense, however, to
use codeine and morphine concurrently

■ Hyoscine 0.3–0.6 mg q4h IM/SC

■ Explain to family about 'death rattle'

■ *Limited* use of suction
Suction may be more upsetting for the patient than a 'rattle'

Dry cough

■ Suppress cough with a centrally acting antitussive

■ Nebulized bupivacaine 0.25% (25 mg/10 ml)

A Bird nebulizer gives a particle size of 2-10 Å. Give up to 5 ml
q4h. Maximum dose = 30 ml/day. Anaesthesia of the mouth and
pharynx is minimal because of the laminar flow. Often not
acceptable to a patient because of unpleasant taste. The authors
have used nebulized bupivacaine only rarely.

Dyspnoea

Definition

An unpleasant awareness of difficulty in breathing.

Breathlessness — ¨what the patient complains of
Tachypnoea (fast breathing) ⎫
Hyperpnoea (increased depth ⎬ what the doctor measures
of respiration) ⎭

Incidence

All terminal cancer — 50% ⎫
Bronchogenic cancer — 70% ⎬ increases in the final weeks

Relevant Physiology

Respiration is controlled by the respiratory centres in the pons
and medulla. The volume of breathing is determined largely by
chemical stimuli in the blood and the pattern of breathing by
mechanical stimuli in the lungs, relayed in the vagus nerves.
Respiration is also influenced by other factors:

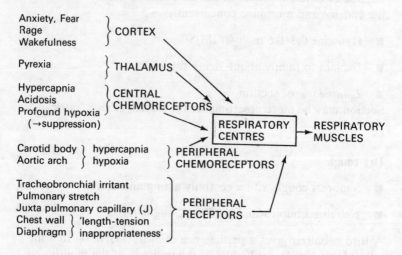

J receptors are stimulated in both pulmonary oedema and
carcinomatous lymphangitis.

Dyspnoea

Patient exacerbates dyspnoea and wastes energy by

■ attempts to improve air exchange
  → increased expiratory effort
  → increased pleural pressure
  → pleural pressure > airway pressure
  → alveolar collapse
  → reduced volume of functioning lung

■ increased respiratory rate
  → relative increase in dead-space ventilation
    decreased tidal volume
    decreased alveolar ventilation
  → increased oxygen demand from increased muscle tension
  and energy expenditure

Respiratory panic attack

In a respiratory panic attack the patient is convinced that he is
suffocating to death.

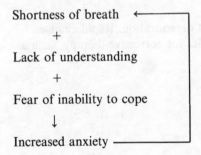

Shortness of breath ←
        +
Lack of understanding
        +
Fear of inability to cope
        ↓
Increased anxiety ─

Causes

Cancer	Debility
Effusion(s)	Anaemia
Obstruction of a main	Atelectasis
bronchus	Pulmonary embolism
Replacement of lung	Pneumonia
by cancer	Empyema
Lymphangitis	
Superior vena caval	*Concurrent*
obstruction	Chronic obstructive
Pericardial effusion	pulmonary disease (COPD)
Massive ascites	Asthma
Abdominal distension	Heart failure
	Acidosis
Treatment	
Pneumonectomy	
Radiation-induced fibrosis	
Chemotherapy:	
bleomycin	
adriamycin	

- A dyspnoeic patient is always an anxious patient
- Dyspnoea is often caused by multiple factors

Assessment

Determine cause of any recent deterioration. Rapid changes commonly present opportunities for corrective therapy, such as thoracentesis or antibiotics.

Treatment Possibilities

- Explanation

'Will I choke to death?'

'Will I suffocate?'

'Will I stop breathing if I go to sleep?'

- Treat reversible causes
  - infection — antibiotic, physiotherapy
  - bronchospasm — bronchodilator
  - cardiac failure — diuretic, digoxin
  - anaemia — blood transfusion
  - pyrexia — antipyretic
  - lymphangitis — corticosteroid
  - obstructed bronchus — corticosteroid, radiation therapy
  - pleural effusion — thoracentesis, pleuradesis
  - ascites — abdominocentesis, diuretics
  - pericardial effusion — paracentesis, corticosteroid

- Non-drug measures
  - a calming presence
  - cool draught (open window, fan)
  - breathing exercises
  - relaxation therapy
  - hypnosis

- Drugs
  - anxiolytic
  - morphine, hydrocodone† (Hycodan) — reduces central respiratory drive
  - nebulized bupivacaine — suppresses J receptors
  - oxygen — corrects hypoxia

- Modify pattern of living
  - help with housework
  - bed downstairs
  - bed rest

Therapeutic Guidelines

Drugs for dyspnoea

- Diazepam: 5–10 mg PO stat and 5–20 mg nocte. In very elderly, 2–5 mg. Reduce dose after several days if drowsy

- Morphine: aim = reduction of respiratory rate to ä comfortable level
  - if on morphine for pain, increase dose by 50%
  - if not on oral morphine, prescribe 5 mg PO q4h; adjust dose upwards as necessary

■ Nebulized bupivacaine 0.25% (25 mg/l0 ml): ultrasound (Pulma-Sonic nebulizer) gives a particle size of 2 Å. This is small enough for bupivacaine to reach the alveoli and the J receptors. Has a possible place in carcinomatous lymphangitis. Often not acceptable to a patient because of unpleasant taste

■ Oxygen: delivered by mask or nasal spectacles. Helpful in *acute* severe dyspnoea. Chronic use should be discouraged because the presence of mask and cylinder leads to increased dependency and anxiety, and further impairment of the patient's quality of life

Respiratory panic attacks

■ Prophylactic education about breathing control

■ A calming presence

■ Oral diazepam 5-l0 mg

Acute tracheal compression/massive haemorrhage into trachea (*very rare*)

■ IV diazepam *or* midazolam until patient unconscious (5–20 mg)

■ PR diazepam *or* IM midazolam 20 mg if IV not possible

■ Continuous company

Noisy tachypnoea in the moribund

■ Although the patient is not aware, other patients become distressed — as does the family. Consider slowing rate down to 10-15/minute with IV diamorphine*/morphine

■ It may be necessary to give 2 or 3 times the previously satisfactory analgesic dose to contain this form of tachypnoea. Aim = reduction of noise by reducing the respiratory rate and decreasing the depth of respiration

Hiccup

Definition

A pathological respiratory reflex characterized by spasm of the diaphragm, resulting in sudden inspiration, and associated with closure of the vocal cords

Causes

- Gastric distension
- Diaphragmatic irritation
- Phrenic nerve irritation
- Brain tumour
- Infection

Treatment

To stop an attack of hiccups

- Reduce gastric distension
  - □ peppermint water (relaxes oesophageal sphincter)
  - □ antiflatulent, e.g. Asilone*, Maalox Plus 10 ml
  - □ metoclopramide, domperidone* 10 mg
  - □ nasogastric intubation

- Pharyngeal stimulation
  - □ drinking from 'wrong' side of a cup
  - □ granulated sugar (2 heaped teaspoons)
  - □ liqueur (2 glasses)
  - □ cold key down back of neck (→ hyperextension of neck)
  - □ nasopharyngeal tube

- Elevation of P_{CO_2}
  - □ breath holding
  - □ rebreathing

- Central suppression of hiccup reflex
  - □ chlorpromazine 25 mg IV if patient distressed and the above measures have failed. Patient should be supine, and warned about drowsiness, possible lightheadedness and palpitations

Maintenance treatment

This depends on the underlying cause.

- Correction of gastric distension
  - Asilone*, Maalox Plus 10 ml *after* meals and bedtime
  - metoclopramide, domperidone 10 mg q4–8h
- Central suppression of hiccup reflex
  - chlorpromazine 10–25 mg t.-q.i.d. PO

This may be necessary when the diaphragm is directly stimulated by tumour

- Suppression of central irritation from intracranial tumour
  - phenytoin 200–300 mg daily
  - valproate sodium 500–1000 mg nocte

Other possible measures

- Benzonatate† (Tessalon perls) 100 mg q.i.d.

- Methylamphetamine 5-10 mg IV

- Phrenic nerve crush — not necessary in terminal care

'Death Rattle'

Definition

A rattling noise produced by the oscillatory movements of secretions, principally in the hypopharynx, in association with the inspiratory and expiratory phases of respiration.

While not pathognomonic of imminent death, the 'death rattle' is generally seen only in patients who are too weak to expectorate effectively.

Treatment Possibilities

- Hyoscine to reduce the production of secretions (see opposite)

- best started sooner rather than later because it does not affect existing secretions
- acts also as a bronchodilator
- has little effect in fulminating pneumonia or left ventricular failure

- Positioning (semi-prone)

- Postural drainage

- Oropharyngeal suction
Most patients dislike suctioning; should generally be reserved for unconscious patients. Use in this circumstance is purely cosmetic, i.e. for the benefit of the relatives, other patients and staff

Hyoscine

Preparations

- Antisecretory
  - sialorrhoea
  - drooling
  - cough
  - 'death rattle'

- Antispasmodic (smooth muscle)
  - intestinal colic
  - bladder spasms
  - rectal tenesmoid pain

- Antiemetic (in obstruction sometimes)

- Anxiolytic-sedative (for moribund)

Limitations

- Anticholinergic effects (see p.102)

- Drowsiness. This is not important in the moribund, in whom it usually produces a peaceful somnolence

- May exacerbate dementia

■ Plasma half-life = 15–40 h; repeated administration leads to cumulation and may result paradoxically in an agitated confusional state. If this occurs, add diazepam *or* midazolam, *or* change to atropine (*Note:* atropine is normally excitatory)

■ Occasionally, acts paradoxically after a single dose; more likely if ≥ 1 mg is given

Preparations

■ SL 0.3 mg (Quick Kwell*)

■ SC/IM 0.4 mg

■ Transdermal (Scopaderm*, Transderm Scop†) 0·5 mg over 3 days

■ Belladonna and opium suppositories (B & O supprettes†) contain about 0.2 mg of belladonna (hyoscine and atropine)

If a SL preparation is required in the USA use *hyoscyamine*, e.g. 0.125 mg (Levsin†). Hyoscyamine is the laevo-isomer of atropine. As the dextro-isomer is virtually inactive, hyoscyamine is approximately twice as potent as atropine

Therapeutic Guidelines

■ Usually given initially in a dose of 0.3–0.4 mg q2–4h. As it cumulates, interval may subsequently be extended

■ Usually *not* possible to extend dose interval when used for 'death rattle'. Dose may need to be increased to 0.6–0.8 mg. In this circumstance, normally given with diamorphine*/morphine

■ Can be used 'as required' for intestinal colic and bladder spasms

7 URINARY SYMPTOMS

Bladder innervation	Hesitancy
Frequency and urgency	Discoloured urine
Bladder spasms	

Bladder Innervation

The urinary bladder has a double innervation:

Innervation	Mediator	Effect	
		Sphincter	Vault
Sympathetic (T10-12,L1)	noradrenaline	contracts (α)	relaxes (β)
Parasympathetic (S2–4)	acetylcholine	relaxes	contracts

When the detrusor muscle contracts, the sphincter relaxes, and vice versa. Anticholinergic drugs not only cause contraction of the bladder neck sphincter but also relax the detrusor muscle.

'you *pee* with your *p*arasympathetics
you *stop* with your *s*ympathetics'

Detrusor muscle sensitivity is

- Increased by prostaglandins

- Decreased by prostaglandin synthetase inhibitors (NSAID)

The external sphincter (urethral) is an additional voluntary mechanism, innervated by the pudendal nerve (S2–4).

The urethra, derived embryologically from the urogenital sinus, is sensitive in the female to oestrogen and progesterone. Idiopathic postmenopausal incontinence is sometimes helped by the prescription of an oestrogen.

Morphine and the Urinary Tract

- Bladder sensation decreased

- Sphincter tone *increased*
- Detrusor tone *increased*
- Ureteric tone and amplitude of contractions increased

In practice, morphine usually has no detectable effect on bladder function. Occasionally, morphine exacerbates hesitancy. In the presence of faecal impaction this may progress to retention. On rare occasions morphine causes urgency, which may lead to urge incontinence.

Frequency and Urgency

Definitions

Frequency

Passage of urine 7+ times during the day and 2+ at night.

Urgency

A strong and sudden desire to void.

Urge incontinence

The involuntary loss of urine associated with a strong desire to void.

Detrusor

The muscle comprising the urinary bladder.

Detrusor instability

Detrusor contracts uninhibitedly and causes:
Diurnal frequency
Nocturnal frequency | increasing severity
Urgency
Urge incontinence

Stress incontinence

The involuntary loss of urine when exercising physically or when coughing, sneezing and laughing.

Genuine stress incontinence

The involuntary loss of urine when the intravesical pressure exceeds the maximum urethral pressure *in the absence of detrusor activity*. The fault always lies in the sphincter mechanism of the bladder, and is associated with multiparity, post-menopause and post-hysterectomy. One or more of the following features will be present

■ Descent of urethro-vesical junction outside intra-abdominal zone of pressure

■ Decrease in urethral pressure due to loss of urethral wall elasticity and contractility

■ Short functional length of urethra

Incidence

The incidence of frequency, urgency and urge incontinence in cancer patients, or in those with urinary tract cancers, is not known.

Frequency is often associated with urgency, which may result in urge incontinence.

The causes of frequency ± urgency overlap with those of urge incontinence.

Causes

Cancer		Concurrent
Intravesical ⎱ mechanical		Infection (cystitis)
Extravesical ⎰ irritation		Idiopathic detrusor
Unrelieved pain		instability
Bladder spasms		Central neurological disease:
Hypercalcaemia — secondary		post cerebral thrombosis
to polyuria		multiple sclerosis
		dementia
Treatment		Uraemia ⎱ secondary
Post-radiation		Diabetes mellitus ⎰ to
Cyclophosphamide cystitis		Diabetes insipidus ⎰ polyuria
Drugs:		
diuretics		
(opioids)		

Urge Incontinence

Urgency sometimes leads to urge incontinence. The precipitating cause is delayed micturition, relative to need. Delay is associated with

- Weakness and difficulty in getting to commode
- Depression ⎫
- Dejection ⎭ disinterest
- Confusion ⎫
- Drowsiness ⎭ lack of awareness

The differential diagnosis includes

- Genuine stress incontinence
- Retention with overflow
- Urinary fistula
- Flaccid sphincter (presacral plexopathy)

Treatment Possibilities

- Explanation
- Treat reversible causes

Cause	Treatment
Diuretic	Reduce or change diuretic
Cystitis	Antibiotic
Sedation	Modify drug regimen

- Non-drug measures
  - □ regular time-contingent voiding (every 1-3 h)
  - □ proximity to toilet
  - □ ready availability of bottle or commode
  - □ rapid response by nurses to patient's request for help
- Anticholinergic drugs
  - □ terodiline* 25–50 mg nocte (plasma half-life = 2.5 days)
  - □ oxybutynin 5 mg q.i.d. (available in UK on 'named patient' basis)
  - □ amitriptyline 25–50 mg nocte (see p. 119)
  - □ propantheline 15 mg b.-t.i.d.

The authors regard these as the drugs of choice for detrusor instability

- Sympathomimetics
  - e.g. terbutaline (Bricanyl) 5 mg t.i.d.
- Musculotropic drugs
  - flavoxate (Urispas) 200–400 mg q.i.d.
- NSAID
  - flurbiprofen 50-l00 mg b.i.d.
  - naproxen 250–500 mg b.i.d.
- Topical analgesic
  - phenazopyridine (Pyridium) l00–200 mg t.i.d.

Bladder Spasms

Definition

Transient deep painful sensations felt mainly in the suprapubic region caused by spasm of the detrusor muscle, most commonly secondary to irritation of the trigone. Variable in frequency and intensity.

Causes

Cancer			*Treatment*
Intravesical	}	irritation	Radiation fibrosis
Extravesical			Indwelling catheter:
Anxiety			without retention
			(mechanical irritation)
Concurrent			with partial retention
Infection (cystitis)			(catheter sludging)
			secondary to infection

Treatment Possibilities

- Explanation
- Treat reversible causes

Cause	Treatment
Infection (cystitis)	Bladder washouts (if catheterized)
	Change indwelling catheter
	Intermittent catheterization q4–6h
	Encourage oral fluids
	Urinary antiseptics[1]:
	hexamine hippurate (Hiprex)
	hexamine mandelate (Mandelamine)
	Antibiotics:
	systemic
	by instillation
Catheter irritation	Change catheter
	Reduce volume of balloon
Catheter sludging	Bladder washouts:
	tap water
	chlorhexidine and benzocaine (Hibitane)
	Noxyflex* ⎫ if cheaper alternative
	Renacidin† ⎭ ineffective
	Continuous bladder irrigation

1 Hexamine effective only in acid urine

- Analgesics to control background pain

- Drugs to reduce detrusor sensitivity
  - ☐ anticholinergic drugs:
    terodiline* 25–50 mg nocte (plasma half-life = 2.5 days)
    oxybutynin 5 mg t.-q.i.d. (available in UK on 'named patient' basis)
    amitriptyline 25–50 mg nocte (see p. 119)
    propantheline 15 mg b.-t.i.d.

The authors regard these as the drugs of choice for bladder spasms
  - ☐ hyoscine (Quick Kwells*) 0.3 mg b.-q.i.d. SL
  - ☐ hyoscyamine (twice as potent as hyoscine):
    Levsin† 0.125 mg b.-q.i.d. SL
    Levsinex Timecaps† (SR) 0.375 mg b.i.d.
    Cystospaz† 0.15 mg b.-q.i.d.
    Cystospaz-M† (SR) 0.375 mg b.i.d.
  - ☐ belladonna and opium suppositories (B & O Supprettes†) up to 1 every hour
    Each B & O Supprette contains either 30 mg (No. 15A) or 60 mg (No. 16A) of powdered opium and approximately 0.2 mg of belladonna alkaloids
  - ☐ flavoxate (Urispas) 100–200 mg t.-q.i.d.
    (a weak detrusor relaxant)

☐ NSAID:
　　flurbiprofen 50-l00 mg b.i.d.
　　naproxen 250–500 mg b.i.d.
☐ phenazopyridine (Pyridium) l00–200 mg t.i.d.
　　(a transitional cell analgesic)
■ Interrupt pain pathways
　☐ coeliac axis plexus block
　☐ lumbar sympathetic block
Both have recently been reported as beneficial in the
management of intractable, distressing bladder pain. The
authors have no personal clinical experience of these measures
in the management of bladder spasm

Hesitancy

Definition

A prolonged delay between attempting to void and achieving
micturition.

Causes

Cancer
Malignant enlargement of
　prostate
Infiltration of bladder neck
Presacral plexopathy
Spinal cord compression

Debility
Loaded rectum
Inability to stand to void
Infection
Generalized weakness

Treatment
Drugs:
　phenothiazines ⎫
　haloperidol ⎪
　cyclizine ⎬ anticholinergic
　antihistamines ⎪ side effects
　tricyclics ⎭
　morphine (occasionally)
Intrathecal nerve block
Surgical damage to bladder innervation

Concurrent
Benign enlargement of prostate

Treatment Possibilities

■ Explanation

■ Treat reversible causes

Causes	Treatment
Anticholinergic drugs	Modify drug regimen if possible
Loaded rectum	Suppositories ⎫ maintenance Enema ⎬ laxative Manual removal ⎭ regimen
Inability to void lying down	Nursing assistance to enable more erect posture
Benign enlargement of prostate	Transurethral resection

■ Drugs

If current drug therapy is probable cause, consider modification rather than introduce an additional drug

■ □ selective α-1 adrenoreceptor antagonist:

prazosin (Hypovase*, Minipress†) 0.5-1 mg b.-t.i.d. — may cause postural hypotension

It is recommended that an initial dose is given in the evening when the patient is lying down. Blood pressure should be taken before and 2 h after the initial dose to gauge the hypotensive effect

□ cholinergic drugs:

bethanichol (Myotonine*, Urecholine†) 10–30 mg b.i.d. may be used in conjunction with an α-adrenergic blocker

□ anticholinesterase:

distigmine* (Ubretid) 5 mg daily-b.i.d.

pyridostigmine (Mestinon) 60-120 mg up to q4h

■ Catheter

Discoloured Urine

There are many causes of discoloured urine. The patient and his family fear that it is evidence of further deterioration. If the urine is red, it is assumed to be haematuria. The following list includes most of the common causes of discolouration.

- Dietary
  - rhubarb → *red*
  - beetroot → *red*

- Drugs
  - adriamycin → *red*
  - danthron (co-danthrusate*) → *red/green/blue*
  - methylene blue (Urised†) → *blue*
    Urised is a combination of urinary antiseptics
    (methenamine, methylene blue, phenylsalicylate, benzoic
    acid) and parasympatholytics (atropine, hyoscyamine)
  - phenazopyridine → *yellow/orange*
    Pyridium (phenazopyridine)
    Azo-Gantanol† (phenazopyridine & sulphamethoxazole)
    Azo-Gantrisin (phenazopyridine & sulfisoxazole)
  - phenolphthalein → *pink* (in alkaline urine) present in
    several proprietary laxatives (e.g. Agarol)

- Infection
  - Pseudomonas aeruginosa (pyocyanin)
    → *blue* (in alkaline urine)

8 SKIN CARE

Pruritus	Decubitus ulcer
Dry skin	Malignant ulcer
Wet skin	

Skin care is generally considered a nursing task. Even so, there
are many occasions when a team approach is of benefit.

Pruritus

Definition

An unpleasant sensation perceived in the skin which provokes an
urge to scratch.

Synonym — itching

Pathophysiology

Pruritus shares neural receptors and pathways with pain. It is the
spatial and temporal pattern of neural excitation which
determines the perceived sensation.

Pruritus is also characterized by its own precipitants, blockers,
potentiators and range of intensity. The cutaneous mediators are
poorly understood. Histamine, by a direct effect on cutaneous
nerves, may mediate itch in urticaria.

Prostaglandins of the E series, believed to be generated in many
inflammatory dermatoses, are not themselves pruritogenic but can
potentiate itch caused by other factors.

Factors which increase the perception of pruritus

- Dehydration

- Heat → vasodilatation

- Proximity to another pruritic area
- Anxiety
- Boredom

Causes

Disorder of skin hydration

- Xerosis (dry flaky skin)
- Wet macerated skin

Primary skin disease

- Scabies
- Pediculosis (lice)
- Allergic contact dermatitis

Common skin allergens to which dying patients are exposed

Neomycin preparations	—	e.g. Cicatrin*, Polybactrin*, Mycolog†
Antihistamine creams		
Local anaesthetic creams	—	but not lignocaine
Alcohol	—	in topical antipruritics and alcohol wipes
Wool wax alcohols	—	in lanolin
Rubber	—	undersheets, elastic pillow coverings, venepuncture equipment
Paraphenylenediamine ⎱ Chromates ⎰	—	in leather restraints

- Atopic dermatitis
- Urticaria
- Bullous pemphigoid
- Dermatitis herpetiformis

Endogenous

- Drug reaction
- Cholestatic jaundice
- Renal failure
- Hodgkin's lymphoma

- Cancer
- Cutaneous metastatic infiltration
- Haematological
  - iron deficiency
  - polycythaemia
- Endocrine
  - thyroid disorders
  - hyperparathyroidism
- Diabetes — usually localized and related to Candidiasis
- Psychiatric

Treatment Possibilities

A dry skin is almost always present in patients with terminal cancer and pruritus, even when there is a definite endogenous cause. As a general rule measures to correct skin dryness should precede, or go hand in hand with, specific measures.

Provided much attention is given to skin care, pruritus is not intractable except occasionally in lymphoma or renal failure.

Optimal skin hydration

- Dry skin (see p. 151)
- Wet skin (see p. 153)

General measures

- Discourage scratching; keep nails cut short; allow gentle rubbing
- Avoid hot, long baths
- Dry skin gently by 'patting' with soft towel
- Avoid overheating and sweating

Topical measures for worst affected areas

- Calamine lotion as required
- Crotamiton (Eurax) cream b.-t.i.d.
This has both mild antipruritic and antiscabetic properties

- Antihistamine containing creams b.-t.i.d., e.g. Anthisan*
  (mepyramine), Caladryl (calamine and diphenhydramine)
  Prolonged use of an antihistamine cream may lead to contact
  dermatitis and increased pruritus. Discontinue if the skin becomes
  inflamed and substitute 1% hydrocortisone cream until settled.

Drugs

- Review medication in case it is partly or mainly the cause
  - associated with drug-induced rash
  - recently prescribed opioid analgesic (rare)

Common cutaneous drug reactions

Morbilliform drug reactions
cephalosporins
danthron
penicillins
phenytoin
sulphonamides

Urticaria-like reactions
cephalosporins
opioids
penicillins
radio-opaque dyes
sulphonamides

Toxic epidermal necrolysis (rare)
allopurinol
penicillin
phenylbutazone
sulphonamides

Phenytoin pseudolymphoma

- Antihistamines, e.g.
  - chlorpheniramine (Piriton) 4 mg b.-t.i.d.
  - promethazine (Phenergan) 25–50 mg nocte
  - trimeprazine (Vallergan) 5–10 mg b.-t.i.d.; 10–30 mg nocte
  - hydroxyzine (Atarax*; Vistaril†) 10–25 mg b.-t.i.d.;
    25–100 mg nocte

The majority of patients with terminal cancer and pruritus never
need an antihistamine if appropriate skin care is undertaken.
An antihistamine without skin care is of little benefit.

■ Consider short-term systemic corticosteroid if skin inflamed as a result of scratching, but not infected e.g.
  □ dexamethasone 2 mg daily
  □ prednisolone 10 mg daily-b.i.d.

Specific measures

■ Androgen in cholestatic jaundice, e.g. stanozolol 5 mg daily *or* methyltestosterone† 25 mg b.i.d. SL
  □ takes 5–7 days to achieve maximum effect
  □ mode of action unknown
  □ may increase jaundice, despite easing pruritus
  □ masculinization usually not a problem

■ Cholestyramine (Questran) 4 g q.i.d. in cholestatic jaundice
  □ theoretically of value but *not* recommended
  □ ill patients find cholestyramine granules difficult to swallow
  □ androgens are easier to take and are more reliable

■ Aspirin *or* alternative NSAID if local pruritus related to cutaneous infiltration by disseminated breast cancer

Dry Skin

Description

Rough, scaly, flaky, hyperkeratotic skin. Can be either fine or coarse in type. A factor in almost all cases of itching in terminal disease except those characterized by wet, macerated skin and secondary infection.

Synonym — xerosis

Pathophysiology

The stratum corneum or keratin layer, the most superficial layer of the skin, needs to be hydrated in order to function as a protective layer.

Water is held in the oil layer secreted by sebaceous glands.

Dried out keratin contracts and splits, exposing the dermis and forming fine scales which flake off.

The exposed dermis becomes inflamed and itchy. Scratching increases inflammation and a vicious circle is created.

The vicious circle is broken only by adding moisture and retaining it, thus enabling reconstitution of the keratin layer.

Treatment Possibilities

General considerations

■ Attention must be paid to the selection of the *vehicle* carrying an active ingredient

■ The vehicle must be a lubricant, either to provide physical occlusion and prevent water evaporation or to bind water chemically to skin

■ The greater the concentration of oil in a lubricant the more wetting power it has

■ Lubricants in decreasing concentration of oil
  □ grease (yellow soft paraffin/petroleum jelly/petrolatum)
  □ ointment
  □ cream (suspension of water in oil)
  □ lotion (suspension of oil in water)

Specific measures

■ Stop using soap — use one of the following instead
  □ emulsifying ointment BP*
  □ non-detergent cleaning bar, e.g. emulsifying wax BP
    4 parts, white soft paraffin 1 part, purified water
    0.555 parts; proprietary preparations are also available
  □ bath emollient, e.g. Oilatum, Alpha Keri, Aveeno Colloidal

■ 'Oil' dry itchy areas after bath and each evening, e.g. lanolin, olive oil, emollient cream (e.g. E45*, Keri-Original†), *oily* Calamine

■ Place a wet cloth over a dry itchy area for 15–20 min and, after removal, apply ointment or cream to keep the skin damp

■ Clioquinol (Vioform)-hydrocortisone cream b.-t.i.d. if inflamed

Wet Skin

Description

Maceration, blisters, exudate, pus (secondary infection).

Pathophysiology

Skin never away from water and never able to dry .

Frequent sites in bedridden patient are those where two layers of skin are apposed:

- □ perineum
- □ between buttocks ⎫
- □ groins ⎬ especially in the incontinent
- □ under breasts ⎭
- □ between fingers — especially if arthritic

Also around ulcers and stomas

Keratin absorbs water and swells → permanent damage and maceration.

Protective barrier broken → infection, usually with yeast, less commonly with staphylococcus and streptococcus → inflammation and pruritus.

Treatment Possibilities

- ■ Protect the skin at risk with an appropriate barrier
  - □ zinc oxide paste where two areas of skin are apposed
  - □ barrier cream e.g. Drapolene* or Desitin†) for legs, backs, arms, around the edges of decubiti and ulcers

Do not use petroleum jelly/petrolatum, ointment or cream under breasts or in groins

- Dry out the skin
  - avoid ointments and creams
  - dry carefully with hair dryer
  - an aqueous solution applied topically alone or as a compress t.i.d. and allowed to dry out completely
    — if not infected use menthol 0.25–1% solution or aluminium acetate (Burows solution)
    — if infected use an antifungal solution (clotrimazole 1%)
    — if very inflamed use 1% cortisone solution for 1–2 days
  - generally avoid adsorbent powders, e.g. starch, talc, zinc oxide — an excess tends to form a hard abrasive coating on the skin

- Monitor for allergic contact dermatitis secondary to topical agents. This may look similar to the initial problem

Decubitus Ulcer

Definition

Ulceration of the skin as a result of extrinsic pressure and shearing forces.

Pathophysiology

The ulceration is due to tissue ischaemia, caused by pressure which is greater than capillary pressure (25 mmHg). This occurs particularly over bony prominences.

When sitting, pressure on skin over ischial tuberosity is about 300 mmHg. Pressure > 70 mmHg for 2 h produces irreversible cellular changes which lead to cell death.

Sites in the terminally ill

Major	Minor
Ear	Occipital
Thoracic spine (apex of kyphosis)	Mastoid
Sacrum	Acromion
Greater trochanter	Spine of scapula
Head of fibula	Lateral condyle of humerus
Malleolus	Ischial tuberosity

Causes

Intrinsic	Extrinsic
Emaciation	Pressure
Diminished mobility	Shearing forces
Tissue fragility	Trauma
Anaemia	Friction
Blood dyscrasia	Crumpled bedclothes
Malnutrition:	Restraints
protein	Bedrails
vitamin C	Infection
zinc deficiency	Moisture
Diabetes mellitus	Poor hygiene
Poor peripheral perfusion	
Incontinence	
Neurological deficit:	
motor	
sensory	
Old age	
Restlessness	
Obtundation	

Staging of Decubitus Ulcers

There is no universally agreed classification for decubitus ulcers; most include pre-ulcer erythema.

Stage 1A Blanching erythema ⎫
Stage 1B Non-blanching erythema ⎬ skin not broken
Stage 2   Superficial skin loss (graze) ⎫
Stage 3   Blister and eschar formation ⎪
Stage 4   Clean ulcer with red granulating base ⎬ skin broken
Stage 5   Infected ulcer or grey slough in base ⎭

Prevention

Pressure redistribution

- Mattresses
  - water-filled camping bed, e.g. Lilo*, Sears camping mattress† (see next page)
  - air bed, e.g. Roho, Ripple, Kinair , Mediscus†
  - water bed
  - Clinitron bed — this reduces skin pressure to <25 mmHg, i.e. less than capillary pressure
  This is the only bed on which a patient does not need turning

- Wheelchair — inflatable cushion (Roho) or eggcrate foam
Shift weight every 15 min if arms strong enough

- Sheepskin mats, elbow and heel pads

- Pillows

- Flannel blankets

- Bed cradles

- Reposition patient by turning
Time interval dependent on observed rate of erythema formation

- Self-adhering urethane foam (3M Reston Foam†)

Use of a camping mattress (Lilo*, Sears†) as a water bed

- Fill with water at body temperature instead of air

- Correct buoyant flotation is most important. When the patient lies on the mattress, top and bottom surface should not meet at any point. Conversely, the mattress should not present a hard surface because of overfilling

- The bed is made with normal sheets, taking care not to tuck in too tightly

- The bedridden patient will maintain the water temperature. This is different from a commercial water bed which must be heated because of the much greater volume of water

- Heat is retained by an electric blanket or heating pad when the patient is out of bed. The electric blanket is not used when the patient is in bed

- When filled, the camping mattress weighs about 120 kg. Thus it can be used in the home where floors are often unable to withstand the weight of a commercial water bed. If used in hospital, the bed can be moved in order to enable the patient to attend concerts and other social events

- Mattresses are washed with a germicide before re-use

- Holes are mended with a puncture repair kit.

Skin care

- Inspection at each change of position
  - □ erythema lasting > 30 min = Stage 1A
  - □ enlist patient and family help

- Optimal hydration and hygiene
  - □ dry skin (see p. 151)
  - □ wet skin (see p. 153)

- Avoidance of trauma
  - □ *no* restraints or bedrails
  - □ patients lifted for movement and turning, not dragged
  - □ loose clothing, smooth bedding
  - □ avoid overheating or sweating
  - □ non-adhesive tape for dressings
  - □ keep nails cut short

Nutrition

- Goals have to be modified in the dying patient

- Plasma albumin concentration ideally > 30 g/L (3 g/100 ml) and haemoglobin > 10 g/100 ml

- Dietary supplements
  - □ vitamin C 500 mg/day
  - □ zinc, if plasma zinc < 100 μg/100 ml (see p. 160)
    The authors rarely consider this option

Treatment Guidelines

Common conditions that delay healing are

- Tissue hypoxia

- Necrotic ulcer surface

- Infection

- Inappropriate care

- Physical debility and immobilization

An ulcer will not heal without an adequate blood supply. Local pressure must therefore be avoided at all times in an established ulcer.

Growth of clean red granulation tissue can occur only after the elimination of local infection and necrotic tissue (eschar).

Granulation tissue must be protected from reinfection, drying out and trauma particularly when the dressing is changed.

Antiseptics do not produce sterile ulcers. The aim is to decrease the quantity of bacteria and to eliminate pathogens, e.g. anaerobic bacteria, Pseudomonas aeruginosa, Klebsiella and Providencia, because these delay healing.

Stage 1A (blanching) and 1B (non-blanching erythema)

■ Pressure relief — no pressure until erythema has resolved
  □ 4 h or less in stage 1A
  □ 48 h in stage 1B

■ Surface treatment
  □ avoid rubbing
  □ expose to air — if macerated, dry with hair dryer

Stage 2 (superficial skin loss; graze)

■ Pressure relief

■ Surface treatment — cover with a semipermeable membrane, e.g. Opsite, Tegaderm, Bioclusive*, Second Skin†

Stage 3 (closed blister or eschar)

■ Pressure relief

■ Surface treatment
  □ keep fluid bleb intact — cover with semipermeable membrane (see above)
  □ eschar — if no infection, pain-free and prognosis <4 weeks, leave intact; otherwise, remove eschar with scalpel bit by bit

Stage 4 (clean ulcer; red granulating base)

■ Pressure relief

- Surface treatment
  - clean with antiseptic :
    povidone-iodine 10% (Betadine)
    oxychlorosene 0.1–0.5% (Clorpactin)
    sodium hypochlorite (Zonite†)
  - Granuflex*, Duoderm† dressing — an outer waterproof polyurethane foam bonded to a matrix of hydrocolloid particles and a hydrophobic polymer. The hydrocolloid particles absorb exudate and swell to form a soft moist gel inside the wound cavity. When removed, some gel remains on the wound bed so that delicate granulation tissue is undisturbed. The gel can, however, be washed away with saline
- Consider surgery if prognosis > 6 months

Stage 5 (infected ulcer or grey slough in base)

- Pressure relief
- Surface treatment
  - wet-to-dry dressings with antiseptic (see above)
  - desloughing agent (Aserbine*, Elase†, Ananase†) — not often necessary
    use if eschar too soggy for surgical debridement and does not debride easily with wet-to-dry dressings

Desloughing agents cause maceration of normal skin and should be used with great care

- Systemic antibiotic only if surrounding cellulitis
  - metronidazole
  - clindamycin

Systemic antibiotics encourage overgrowth of resistant organisms

Therapeutic Considerations

- Natural sheepskin is preferable to synthetic alternatives but is harder to look after

- Bandor adsorbent dressings are very useful to control malodour; they are expensive but can be washed, sterilized and re-used

■ All adherent tapes, including the hypoallergenic variety, can blister and denude fragile skin. They must not be placed under tension

■ The daily zinc requirement is 15 mg/day. If correcting a deficiency, prescribe zinc sulphate monohydrate 61.8 mg (zinc 22.5 mg) capsules* (Z Span) *or* zinc gluconate (zinc 10 mg) capsules† *or* lozenges† (Orazinc) daily-b.i.d.

■ Most other zinc sulphate preparations are 200–220 mg. If using these, the plasma zinc concentration must be monitored because toxic levels are easily achieved, particularly in renal failure.

Malignant Ulcer

Definition

A skin ulcer associated with a superficial primary or secondary cancer.

The main goal of treatment is the prevention of malodour because this leads to isolation of the patient and social ostracism.

Treatment Possibilities

■ Gauze soaked in adrenaline (epinephrine) 1:1000 will reduce capillary bleeding — use only when healing is not a goal

■ Irrigation of ulcer with hydrogen peroxide 3%

■ Local antiseptic (see p. 159)

■ Adsorbent dressing (Bandor, Actisorb)

■ Air freshener (Nilodor; electric deodorizer)

■ Systemic antibiotics (metronidazole, clindamycin)

■ If the above measures fail to prevent malodour, pack the ulcer with benzoyl peroxide 10–20%.

- benzoyl peroxide is a powerful organic oxidizing agent
- it often produces an irritant dermatitis and may cause a contact allergic dermatitis
- normal skin surrounding the ulcer must be protected with petroleum jelly/petrolatum or zinc oxide paste
- a large cavity or an undercut margin is firmly packed with surgical gauze soaked with benzoyl peroxide, so as to obtain good contact with the walls of the cavity
- a dressing is cut from sterile terry towelling to fit the ulcer exactly and saturated with benzoyl peroxide. It may be applied directly to a shallow ulcer surface or over the surgical gauze packing when there is a large cavity. This dressing must not overlap normal skin
- plastic film is placed over the dressing (Clingfilm*, Saran Wrap†) and allowed to adhere to the ointment protecting the surrounding normal skin
- an abdominal pad dressing is taped over the plastic film with hypoallergenic tape (Dermacel, 3M)
- unless there is excessive exudate, dressing may need to be changed only once a day
- exudate must be cleansed from the wound surface with saline at each change of dressing
- occasionally a patient may complain of burning in the ulcer while the dressing is being changed. This subsides within 30 min

9 LYMPHOEDEMA

Lymphoedema
Management strategy
Skin care
Exercise

Massage
Intermittent pneumatic
compression

Lymphoedema

Definition

An accumulation of lymph in the interstitial space of subcutaneous tissue. It results from a disturbance of the equilibrium between the transport capacity of the clearing system and the load of lymph to be cleared. In cancer, most commonly, one limb is affected and sometimes the adjacent quadrant of the trunk as well.

Causes

- Surgery and/or radiotherapy to the axilla or groin

- Postoperative infection

- Axillary, groin or intra-pelvic recurrence

Symptoms

- Tightness (tissue swelling and stretching of the skin)

- Discomfort or pain secondary to
  □ associated venous obstruction
  □ myoligamentous strain caused by increased limb weight
  □ inflammation and infection
  □ psychological distress

Limb Signs

■ Persistent swelling of part or whole of limb — non-pitting if extensive interstitial fibrosis

■ Deepening of skin folds

■ Hyperkeratosis

■ Stemmer's sign, i.e. an inability to pick up a fold of skin at the base of a digit

The absence of this sign does not, however, necessarily exclude lymphoedema

Trunk Signs

■ If the axillary fold shows signs of oedema it may be assumed that the adjacent trunk is involved. The lymphoedema may be visible, e.g. underwear may leave deeper markings on the affected side

■ A fold of skin should be pinched up simultaneously on both sides on the trunk. If lymphoedema is present, the skin is more difficult to pinch up. Radiotherapy, however, also causes subcutaneous thickening

Measurement

■ The *circumference* of the mid-hand, wrist, forearm and upper arm (or mid-foot, ankle, mid-calf and mid-thigh) should be measured

■ The forearm and upper arm (or calf and thigh) should be measured at a fixed number of cm above and below the olecranon (or tibial tuberosity)

Management Strategy

As lymphoedema cannot be cured, the aim is to achieve maxim? improvement and long-term control. The earlier treatment is started the easier it is to achieve a good result. Treatment comprises

- Explanation
- Skin care
- Exercise
- Containment hosiery
- Massage

Success requires full cooperation. To this end, the patient needs *information* about the condition and *encouragement* to become self-sufficient in the daily management of the swollen limb. Doctors, nurses, physiotherapists and occupational therapists can all help in this.

Diuretics are of limited value in the treatment of pure lymphoedema unless

- The swelling has developed or deteriorated since the prescription of a corticosteroid or NSAID

- There is a cardiac or venous component

Intensive Treatment

The following are indications for intensive treatment with compression bandaging and/or intermittent pneumatic compression

- Grossly oedematous limb (i.e. severe lymphoedema)

- Awkwardly shaped limb (e.g. very deep skin folds)

- Involvement of fingers

- Involvement of trunk

- Persistent copious lymphorrhoea (lymph leakage)

- Persistent severe pain

- Recurrent acute inflammatory episodes

A description of the use of compression bandaging is beyond the scope of this book but may be found in Badger C and Twycross R 1988 *Management of Lymphoedema*. Available from Sir Michael Sobell House, Oxford.

Skin Care

Chronic lymphoedema leads to changes in both subcutaneous tissue and skin. The protein in lymph causes fibrosis and thickening. The skin tends to become dry and warty.

Static lymph makes the limb vulnerable to infection. Even a small break in the skin enables bacteria to gain access to an ideal growth medium. Infection stimulates fibrosis and leads to scarring of the lymphatics. Careful hygiene reduces the risk of infection. After washing, the swollen limb should be dried carefully, paying particular attention to between the digits.

Oil or a 'moisturizing' cream should be applied to prevent drying and cracking. Apply at night so that it is fully absorbed before containment hosiery is put on in the morning. Any bland hand cream or body lotion will do; the important thing is to apply it daily.

Avoid perfumed creams or lotions as they may cause irritation.

Acute Inflammatory Episodes

■ Static protein-rich lymph may cause low-grade inflammation. It responds to measures aimed at relieving the oedema

■ A hot red tender area accompanied by a rapid increase in swelling suggests infection. This should be treated promptly with rest, elevation and antibiotics (see opposite)

■ Fungal infections are common, e.g. tinea pedis. They should be treated with an appropriate anti-fungal agent

■ For patients who have repeated episodes of infection, long-term prophylaxis is the best way of preventing recurrent attacks and minimizing infection-exacerbated fibrosis

Antibiotic treatment for limb infection in obstructive lymphoedema

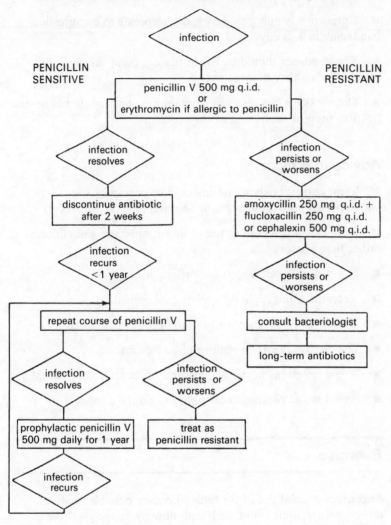

Ulceration

■ This occurs only if there is a combined lymphovenous disorder or if there are cutaneous tumour deposits

■ Since the presence of oedema delays healing, containment hosiery or bandages should be used with appropriate dressings

Lymphorrhoea

■ Cutaneous lymph leakage usually responds to compression bandaging in 1–2 days

■ The bandages should be left in place around the clock but replaced when they become wet

■ Once leakage has resolved, containment hosiery should be fitted to prevent recurrence of the problem

Advice to Patients

■ Treat cuts, scratches, and insect bites promptly. Clean well and apply an antiseptic cream or solution (e.g. Savlon, TCP)

■ Take care when cutting toe or finger nails; use nail clippers rather than scissors

■ Dry well between fingers/toes after washing

■ Keep the skin supple by applying oil or bland cream

■ Do not allow the swollen limb to become sunburned

■ Use electric razors to remove unwanted hair

■ Avoid injections in the swollen arm, including blood sampling

■ Avoid blood pressure measurements on the swollen arm

Exercise

Encourage normal use of the limb whenever possible because muscle contractions stimulate lymph flow by 'massaging' the overlying tissues. Exercise also helps to prevent stiff joints.

Excessive exercise, however, can be harmful because it induces vasodilatation and increases lymph production. Accordingly, patients should avoid carrying heavy objects.

Specific exercises have two aims

■ Putting joints through a full range of movements

■ Using forearm/calf muscles to improve lymph drainage

If active movements are impossible, passive exercises should be carried out at least twice a day.

Well-fitting containment hosiery should be worn during exercise.

Elevation is of Limited Value

■ While it makes sense to elevate a swollen limb when resting, it is better to encourage movement rather than set aside a specific time for elevation

■ Patients with leg oedema should avoid standing or sitting with dependent legs for long periods

■ Maximum benefit is achieved by elevation to the level of the heart. In pure lymphoedema, the use of containment hosiery generally obviates the need for elevation

Avoid Slings

■ Immobilizing a swollen arm allows fluid to pool in a limb and can lead to fixed shoulder and elbow joints

■ If the arm is grossly swollen and its weight makes walking difficult, the answer is to reduce the oedema

■ If the patient's prognosis is so poor that attempts to reduce the size of the arm are considered inappropriate, a sling can be used when the patient is walking. It should, however, be removed when the patient is at rest, and the arm supported on pillows preferably in an extended position

■ A paralysed arm is an indication for a sling when walking

Massage

Massage is used to stimulate contraction of the skin lymphatics which are usually undamaged. This 'milking' action improves superficial lymph drainage.

Massage can be done manually or by using an electrical body massager, e.g. Pifco or Clairol.

All lymphoedema patients benefit from massage. Massage is the only way of clearing oedema from the trunk. Clearing the trunk enhances drainage from the limb.

If the axillary fold shows signs of oedema it should be assumed that the trunk is involved.

Technique

- The area to be massaged should be bare and the patient lying down. Cream or oil should not be applied as these reduce contact between hand and skin

- Massage starts in a normal area and moves distally into the swollen area. The increase in lymphatic contractions enhances lymph flow out of affected areas and into cleared areas

- The flat of the hand is used to massage and the strokes are firm enough so that the skin moves but not so firm as to mark or redden the skin

- When the front has been treated, the patient should turn over and the back massaged in the same way. Massage of the trunk and limb takes about 20 minutes

- If an electrical body massager is used then the same technique applies. Use at the lowest setting. If the massager comes with a choice of heads, the 'dimpled' head should be used

Intermittent Pneumatic Compression

Pneumatic compression consists of an inflatable sleeve connected to a motor driven air pump. The limb is inserted into the sleeve which inflates and deflates cyclically.

There is a variety of makes (e.g. Flowtron, Talley, Lymphapress, Jobst) and a variety of models. These range from small portable pumps with a single chamber sleeve to larger models with multi-chamber sleeves which inflate and deflate sequentially.

The smaller models usually operate on a predetermined inflation/deflation cycle whereas the larger models offer a selection of cycle times. The machines have a pressure dial which may range from 20 mmHg to as high as 300 mmHg.

The ripple effect of a multi-chamber sequential pump (e.g. Talley

Multicom) is much more effective at shifting fluid than the simple squeezing effect of single-chamber pumps.

Single-chamber pneumatic compression has no direct effect on lymph flow; it simply forces fluid out of the limb via tissue planes and veins.

Multi-chamber pneumatic compression provides additional benefits. The sequential action

■ Stimulates superficial lymph flow

■ Possibly helps to disrupt tissue fibrosis

If external support is not fitted *between* treatment sessions, fluid will seep back into the over-stretched tissues.

Compression pumps should be used for a total of 4 h/day for 2 weeks.

Use the highest pressure that the patient finds comfortable up to 60 mmHg. Pressures higher than this may result in the obstruction of blood flow, increased venous leakage and increased lymph production.

Indications

The use of a compression pump speeds up the rate of improvement; it does not normally lead to a better result.

■ Only a minority of patients need pneumatic compression

■ Compression pumps are useful in the initial intensive phase of limb reduction, particularly if there is extensive fibrosis

Contraindications

■ Extensive cutaneous metastases around upper arm and shoulder

■ Trunk oedema (fluid from limb is simply pushed from the limb to an already congested area)

■ Infection (it is too painful)

■ Venous thrombosis (may dislodge a recently formed thrombus; delay pneumatic compression for 2 months)

PART TWO

10 ORAL MORPHINE IN ADVANCED CANCER

Oral morphine
Response to morphine
Starting treatment with morphine
Coping with unwanted effects
More questions about morphine
Other important uses of morphine

Oral Morphine

1 What are the indications for morphine in advanced cancer?

Main	*Subsidiary*
Pain	Cough
Dyspnoea	Diarrhoea

The use of morphine to help dyspnoea is discussed in sections 61 and 62.

Note: Sedation only is *not* an indication for morphine.

2 Why use morphine? What about other strong opioids?

Morphine is a versatile drug. Orally, it has a plasma half-life of 2–2.5 h and, apart from patients with renal failure, there is no danger of drug cumulation. By mouth, no other strong opioid shows a clear advantage over morphine.

Papaveretum (strong opium), oxycodone† and hydromorphone† are essentially morphine 'look-alikes'. Levorphanol and phenazocine* have longer plasma half-lives and generally need to be given only q6–8h; and methadone only q8–12h. Both levorphanol and methadone tend to cumulate when administered regularly. Thus, a patient may become drowsy and muddled unless the dose is reduced or given less frequently.

Cumulation appears not to be a problem with phenazocine*. It is available, however, only in 5 mg tablets. This is equivalent to 20–25 mg of oral morphine and many patients do not need as much as this.

3 What is the best way of giving morphine by mouth?

In practice, the choice lies between a solution of morphine sulphate/hydrochloride ('aqueous morphine') and SR tablets. Aqueous morphine has to be administered *every 4 hours*; SR tablets *every 12 hours*. Proprietary preparations of both formulations are available

- ■ Aqueous solution
  - □ Oramorph*
  - □ Roxanol†

- ■ SR tablets
  - □ MST-Continus*, MS Contin†
  - □ Roxanol SR†

Many pharmacies, however, still produce their own aqueous morphine.

At some centres, SR tablets are considered the formulation of choice while at others aqueous morphine is preferred. When cost is an overriding consideration, aqueous morphine should be used. On the other hand, the convenience of a b.i.d. regimen compared with q4h makes the SR form an attractive option, especially for the more active and for those at home.

Initial dose titration with aqueous morphine is recommended, particularly for patients with difficult-to-control pain. At some centres, however, SR tablets are used throughout.

Response to Morphine

4 In relation to pain, when should morphine be used?

From a therapeutic point of view, pain in cancer can be divided into three categories

■ Morphine responsive, i.e. pain that is relieved by morphine

■ Morphine semi-responsive, i.e. pain that is best relieved by the concurrent use of morphine *and* an adjuvant drug

■ Morphine resistant pain, i.e. pain that is not relieved by morphine but may be eased by other drugs

For morphine responsive pains, morphine should be prescribed when codeine (*or* dextropropoxyphene *or* dihydrocodeine*) fails to relieve the patient's pain. The weak opioid should have been administered q4–6h in conjunction with a non-opioid (i.e. aspirin *or* paracetamol/acetaminophen) and appropriate non-drug measures.

Although morphine responsive, functional gastrointestinal pains should be treated more specifically

■ Gastric distension   — dietary advice; antiflatulent
■ Spastic colon   — antispasmodic; bulk-forming drug
■ Constipation   — enema; laxative

These are morphine responsive pains for which morphine should not be used.

5 Which pains are only semi-responsive to morphine?

■ Bone metastasis

■ Nerve compression

■ Raised intracranial pressure

A partial response calls for adjuvant medication and consideration of non-drug treatments

■ Bone pain
  □ NSAID
  □ radiation therapy (treatment of choice)

■ Nerve compression
  □ corticosteroid
  □ neurolytic block (sometimes)

- Raised intracranial pressure
  - corticosteroid
  - use 3–4 pillows (sometimes)

6 What do you mean by 'morphine resistant' pains?

Not all pains respond to morphine. The following pains should be regarded as *morphine resistant*

- Headache
  - tension
  - migraine
- Muscle spasm
- Deafferentation (see p. 34)
- Sympathetic maintained (see p. 36)

Alternative treatments are indicated for these pains. For example, an antidepressive and/or an anticonvulsant for deafferentation pain.

Movement-induced pain is frequently morphine resistant. So much morphine is required for control during activity that the patient becomes unacceptably drowsy at rest. The dose of morphine is therefore balanced against rest pain rather than movement-induced pain.

7 Are there any other important morphine resistant pains?

There are a number of other circumstances in which pain *appears* to be morphine resistant. These include

- Underdosing
  - dose too small
  - dose too infrequent
  - dose given 'as required'
- Poor absorption from the alimentary tract (rare)
- Ignoring emotional, spiritual and social factors

The pain from superficial bedsores also is only semi-responsive to morphine. Here, care in movement plays an important role in management.

8 Can psychological factors really inhibit the action of morphine?

Morphine (or any other opioid) should be given only within the context of comprehensive biopsychosocial care. If psychological factors are ignored, pain may well prove intractable.

A 55-year-old man with recently diagnosed cancer of the oesophagus was still in pain despite receiving SR morphine tablets, *6000 mg* (100 mg x 60) b.i.d. Following inpatient admission to a hospice, he became pain-free on *30 mg* b.i.d. and diazepam 10 mg nocte. He returned home, converted the spare bedroom into a workshop, and was able to spend many happy hours there. The key to success was *listening, explaining* and *setting positive rehabilitation goals*.

The first step is to break the vicious circle of pain, sleeplessness, exhaustion, increasing pain and agitation. Achieving a good night's sleep may require a night sedative or anxiolytic *and* morphine, at least initially.

If the patient is clinically depressed, an antidepressive should be considered. It is, however, not easy initially to distinguish between exhaustion (because of pain and sleeplessness) and depression. With morphine responsive pain, lack of success with morphine combined with an anxiolytic or night sedative is one pointer to depression.

9 Can I ever be confident that the use of morphine will result in complete relief?

Yes — if the pain is morphine responsive. Relief, however, is not an 'all or none' phenomenon. The partial relief obtained with a weak opioid or when morphine is first prescribed often indicates whether the pain is morphine responsive.

Dr: 'When you take your tablets (weak opioid), how soon do you get relief?'

Pt: 'After 20–30 minutes.'

Dr: 'How long does the relief last?'

Pt: 'About one and a half to two hours.'

Dr: 'How much of the pain is relieved by the tablets? 25%, 50%, 75%?

Pt: 'I would say about 50%: they make it bearable.'

Dr: 'That's good, because it tells me that you have a pain that responds to this type of pain-killer. What we have to do now is to find something that is stronger so as to get rid of at least 95% of your pain.

In this situation, the doctor can be confident that the use of morphine will achieve much greater—possibly complete— relief.

Starting Treatment with Morphine

10 What are the basic principles governing the use of morphine in advanced cancer?

- If the pain is morphine resistant do not use morphine

- If the pain is morphine semi-responsive, an adjuvant drug or a non-drug treatment will also be necessary

- Use in context of comprehensive biopsychosocial care

- Administer 'by the mouth'

- Administer 'by the clock'

- Adjust the dose to individual need

- Anticipate and treat vomiting and constipation

- Monitor response

11 How do I decide on the initial dose of oral morphine?

For most patients, 10 mg q4h or SR morphine tablets 30 mg q12h is the correct starting dose. This assumes that they have been taking a weak opioid analgesic regularly but with poor response, or that there was an initial good response followed more recently by less benefit: 'My body seems to have got used to the tablets, doctor.'

If the weak opioid has been taken only t.-q.i.d. 'as required' and has given good, though intermittent, response, the first step may be not to prescribe morphine but to increase the frequency to q4h *regularly*. If the patient is completely pain-free the next day, the regular use of the weak opioid q4h should be continued: *morphine is not indicated*. If the patient is only 75–90% comfortable, treatment with morphine should be started.

12 What about the patient who is taking an alternative strong opioid analgesic?

All strong opioids should be regarded as alternatives to morphine and can be expected to substitute effectively for morphine in the appropriate dose. The important exceptions to this rule are

- Buprenorphine (a partial agonist)

- Pethidine/meperidine

Both buprenorphine and pethidine/meperidine have an analgesic 'ceiling' above which no further benefit is obtained. The ceiling for SL buprenorphine is 3–5 mg a day. This is equivalent to a total daily dose of 180–300 mg of oral morphine

With pethidine/meperidine the ceiling is related to unwanted effects (tremor, twitching, fits, agitation) caused by the accumulation of a toxic metabolite, norpethidine/normeperidine. Thus, it is not possible to use regular oral doses of more than 300 mg. In some patients, particularly those with poor renal function, toxic manifestations occur with much lower doses.

In relation to the other strong opioids, if the patient has been well pain-controlled but is now 'getting used to the tablets', it may simply be necessary to increase the dose in order to regain control.

A decision to change to morphine may be made because

- Of unacceptable drowsiness (sometimes prominent with levorphanol and methadone) *or*

- The drug has to be given q2–3 h because it is short-acting, e.g. pethidine/meperidine and dextromoramide*

13 Is 10 mg of aqueous morphine the right starting dose for a patient previously receiving an alternative strong opioid?

No! If 10 mg of aqueous morphine (or 30 mg of SR morphine) is prescribed in these circumstances, the patient will soon be in severe pain. This is unnecessary, and serves simply to damage the morale of patient and family. It may also result in the potentially dangerous attitude: 'Morphine is no good for Mr Smith's pain: it doesn't work for him.'

This is relevant in the USA where oxycodone† is widely used in combination with a non-opioid — Percodan, Percocet and Tylox. These contain about 5 mg of oxycodone† together with either aspirin or paracetamol/acetaminophen. It is not always appreciated that oxycodone† is a strong opioid equipotent with morphine.

14 What is the right starting dose for patients changing from an alternative strong opioid?

The dose of morphine to be prescribed is calculated as follows

■ Add up the total dose in mg of the alternative strong opioid taken in an average 24 h period

■ Multiply this by the potency of the strong opioid in question (see table below). This is the *total daily dose of morphine* that will give a comparable degree of comfort.

■ If the patient has been in pain despite the use of the alternative strong opioid, the total daily dose of morphine should be increased by about 50%.

■ If using aqueous morphine divide this by 6 and 'round up' to the nearest convenient 5 mg or 10 mg. This is the correct 'q4h' starting dose of morphine. This may be 60 mg or even more

■ If using SR tablets, divide by 2 and 'round up' to the nearest convenient b.i.d. dose. This may be as much as 200 mg

---

Approximate oral opioid potency ratios

pethidine/meperidine	$\frac{1}{8}$	methadone	$3–4^2$
dipipanone*	$\frac{1}{2}$	levorphanol	5
papaveretum	$\frac{2}{3}$	phenazocine*	5
morphine sulphate	1	hydromorphone†	6
oxycodone†	1	buprenorphine*	60^3
dextromoramide*	2^1		

---

1 Dextromoramide — a single 5 mg dose is equivalent to morphine 15 mg (diamorphine* 10 mg) in terms of peak effect but is shorter acting. The overall potency ratio has been adjusted accordingly.

2 Methadone — a single 5 mg dose is equivalent to morphine 7.5 mg (diamorphine* 5 mg). It has a prolonged plasma half-life which leads to accumulation when given repeatedly. This means that when given regularly it is several times more potent .

3 Refers to SL route. In the USA buprenorphine is available only as an injection.

15 Overwhelming pain

Some patients present a picture of 'It's all pain, doctor.' They are usually highly anxious, demoralized, depressed, and exhausted from pain-related insomnia. In this situation there is no way of estimating what a patient will need to achieve relief.

Generally an anxiolytic (diazepam) and morphine need to be prescribed concurrently. The nurse(s) should be instructed to repeat the initial combined medication after 1 h unless the patient is very much more comfortable. Review by the doctor after 2 h and 4 h is not excessive. Subsequent doses of both drugs depend on the initial response.

Overwhelming pain is usually the result of weeks or months of unrelieved severe pain. *It should be regarded as a medical emergency*. Best results are obtained if *one doctor* (or at most two) accepts responsibility for frequent review and prescribing.

16 How soon should a patient be reassessed after commencing aqueous morphine?

Ideally after 2 h and again after 4 h. This is rarely possible if the patient is at home. Monitoring progress must be seen as a team responsibility. The team comprises the patient, family, nurse(s) and doctor. Provided that each one knows his or her part, it is unlikely that anything will go seriously wrong.

The patient and family should be advised that the starting dose may not completely control the pain

■ 'If the morphine is less effective than your old medication, 'top up' with a dose of the old and increase the next dose of morphine solution from 10 ml to 15 ml.'
or

■ 'If the morphine solution is less effective than your old medication, take another dose after 2 h and increase the next regular dose from 10 ml to 15 ml.'
or

■ 'If your pain is not 90% controlled by this time tomorrow, increase the dose of morphine solution from 10 ml to 15 ml.'

In addition, the following general advice should be given:

■ 'If you are unhappy about anything concerning the new

medication, contact me at ... (name and telephone number of doctor or nurse)'

or

■ 'I (or nurse) will be in touch later today/tomorrow to review progress'

or

■ 'Would you phone me tomorrow at ... to let me know how things are going?'

Further, if an unknown team member is scheduled to be on duty, give the patient the name of the person available and a few words of introduction and reassurance:

■ 'Dr X/Nurse Y is on call tonight. We work closely together, and I will tell him/her about you before I leave the office'

It should be exceptional for a patient not to be visited on the second day of treatment by either a doctor or nurse familiar with morphine administration.

During the first few days, it is often necessary to adjust the dose of morphine.

The patient and family usually have many questions they wish to ask about the regular use of morphine: 'Won't I become addicted?' etc. Professional time must be made for such discussion.

Personal professional support is necessary to encourage the patient and family during the period of initial unwanted effects. Also, only the trained professional can recognize when the dose of morphine should be reduced temporarily or when morphine intolerance cannot be circumvented (see section 34).

It is negligent to prescribe morphine and not make arrangements for close supervision by somebody familiar with its use.

17 How soon should the patient become pain-free?

Total immediate success is a bonus. It is best, therefore, to set a series of sequential goals.

■ A good night's sleep free of pain. This will normally be achieved in 2–3 days

■ Comfort at rest (sitting or lying) during the day. This will normally be achieved in 3–5 days

■ Comfort when active. This will normally be achieved in 3–7 days. However, in patients with multiple vertebral or pelvic metastases, this third level of relief may not be possible

■ For patients with persisting activity-precipitated pain, it is necessary to suggest ways in which the patient might modify his pattern of living so as to reduce pain-producing activities

In patients with more than one pain, each pain should be reassessed. Some respond more readily than others. Reassessment remains a continuing necessity. Old pains may get worse and new ones may develop.

If the patient is very anxious or deeply depressed, it may take 3–4 weeks to achieve a satisfactory result.

18   What should be done if the chosen dose of morphine does not adequately or completely relieve the patient's pain?

The aim is to increase the dose progressively until the patient's pain is relieved (dose titration). The patient should be advised to increase the dose by 50% if the first dose is not more effective than the previous medication, or during the second day 'if the pain is not 90% controlled,' even if he feels moderately sleepy.

If the pain is not much relieved after one or two increments, it is possible that the patient has a morphine resistant pain. In this circumstance, an alternative strategy is necessary.

Alternatively, non-relief may indicate that the pain has a higher than average psychological component. This will demand more time, more psychotherapeutic support and probably the prescription of an anxiolytic or an antidepressive.

19   By how much should the dose of morphine be increased?

Generally, a 50% increase is recommended, certainly no less than 33%. Each adjustment takes time and, if an adjustment yields little or no benefit, time and confidence are lost.

It is important to be equally decisive when increasing the dose of SR tablets.

Coping with Unwanted Effects

20 What are the unwanted effects of morphine?

Common unwanted effects of morphine therapy

Initial	*Occasional*
Vomiting	Sweating
Drowsiness	Myoclonic jerks
Unsteadiness	Dry mouth
Confusion	

Continuing	*Late*
Constipation	Depression

Note: 'Addiction' and respiratory depression are *not* listed (see sections 32 and 33).

21 Is the use of morphine limited by unwanted effects?

Generally: No
Occasionally: Yes

Unwanted effects are minimized by close supervision and by the use of an appropriate antiemetic and a laxative.

22 Is an antiemetic always necessary?

If the patient vomits after taking morphine, the morphine will not be absorbed, the patient remains in pain, and confidence in the new medicine is lost. To avoid this, some doctors use an antiemetic routinely whenever morphine is prescribed.

While this is probably good advice for the inexperienced prescriber, once a doctor and the team feel confident in the use of oral morphine, a more discriminatory approach is possible.

The following patients should be prescribed an antiemetic prophylactically

■ Those with current nausea and vomiting.

■ Those who are vomiting as a result of the current use of codeine or other weak opioid

■ Those who have vomited with morphine-like drugs in the past

The following patients need *not* be prescribed an antiemetic prophylactically

■ Those with no current nausea and vomiting

■ Those taking a weak or alternative strong analgesic regularly without nausea or vomiting.

One-third of all patients prescribed morphine never need an antiemetic.

23 Which antiemetic is best?

This depends whether or not morphine is the main or only cause of the vomiting.

Cause	Antiemetic	Usual doses
Drugs ⎫ Biochemical ⎭	haloperidol fluphenazine prochlorperazine	1-3 mg nocte 0.5–2 mg b.i.d. 5 mg q4–8h
Upper bowel (non-obstructive)	metoclopramide domperidone*	10 mg q4–8h 10 mg q4–8h
Intracranial ⎫ Bowel obstruction ⎭	cyclizine meclozine†	50 mg q4–8h 25 mg b.-t.i.d

Haloperidol and fluphenazine are equally good choices for drug-induced nausea and vomiting, and should be used in preference to prochlorperazine.

24 Are there circumstances in which haloperidol or fluphenazine will not control morphine-induced vomiting?

Yes. Although stimulation of the chemoreceptor trigger zone in the brain stem is the commonest cause of morphine-induced vomiting, morphine can precipitate vomiting by other mechanisms

- Delayed gastric emptying
- Secondary to constipation
- Vestibular disturbance

Vomiting secondary to delayed gastric emptying is a real problem in some 5–10% of patients prescribed oral morphine. It is reminiscent of pyloric stenosis. The use of a gastrokinetic antiemetic (i.e. metoclopramide *or* domperidone* 10 mg q4h normally permits the continued use of morphine. If necessary the dose of metoclopramide *or* domperidone* should be increased to 20 mg q4h for a week in the first instance.

Occasionally, it is necessary to consider using two antiemetics concurrently, for example

- Haloperidol with metoclopramide *or* domperidone*
- Haloperidol with cyclizine *or* meclozine†
- Metoclopramide *or* domperidone* with cyclizine *or* meclozine†

Presumably, in these circumstances, there are other emetogenic factors operative, possibly relating to the underlying cancer. In Oxford, less than 10% of cancer patients receiving oral morphine receive two antiemetics concurrently.

25 Can the emetic be stopped?

Vomiting with morphine is mainly an initial unwanted effect. If an antiemetic was prescribed prophylactically, and not to control pre-existing nausea and vomiting, it is good practice to stop it after the patient has been on a steady dose of morphine for a week. Remember that a third of patients receiving morphine never need an antiemetic. If necessary, the emetic can be restarted.

26 Do patients become drowsy on morphine?

Like nausea and vomiting, drowsiness tends to be troublesome during the first 3–7 days, and subsequently should an upward dose adjustment become necessary. Patients should be warned about initial drowsiness and encouraged to persevere in the knowledge that it will lessen after a few days. Occasionally, in the very old and frail patient, it is necessary to reduce the dose of morphine and then increase it again more slowly, every 2–3 days, until adequate relief is obtained.

27   Do some patients go on feeling very drowsy and drugged?

Occasionally, yes (see table below). It is important to distinguish between persistent drowsiness and inactivity or boredom drowsiness. Most patients receiving morphine 'catnap' with ease. This means that they will drop off to sleep if sitting quietly and alone. As many of these patients have little stamina, they need more rest and sleep than when healthy. Provided that they are easily roused and can converse readily when joined by family or friends, continuing inactivity drowsiness should be seen as a bonus. Indeed many patients find that it helps to pass what otherwise might be a long and exhausting day.

If stamina are not limited, the patient can live a normal active life, as any continuing drowsiness is inactivity related.

Checklist for excessive drowsiness in patients receiving oral morphine

---

General factors
Is the patient still recuperating from prolonged fatigue?
Is the patient more ill than I thought?

renal failure	hepatic failure
hypercalcaemia	cerebral metastases
hyponatraemia	septicaemia
hyperglycaemia	cardiac failure
	hypotension

Drug factors
Is the patient completely pain free?

If yes, reduce the dose and review both drowsiness and pain control

Is the patient on a psychotropic drug — notably a benzodiazepine (e.g. diazepam) *or* a phenothiazine (e.g. chlorpromazine)? Is it necessary?

If no, cut it out
If yes, can the dose be reduced?

If the patient is taking a phenothiazine antiemetic, can it be changed to haloperidol *or* metoclopramide?

Patients with renal failure are particularly likely to become drowsy because of cumulation of the active metabolite, morphine-6-glucuronide. This necessitates a reduction in dose of morphine.

Moderate hepatic insufficiency does *not* affect the metabolism of morphine; severe hepatic failure may.

28 Do patients become confused?

Yes, a few. Particularly the elderly who are more sensitive to the effects of morphine. It may be necessary, therefore, to titrate the dose of morphine more slowly in these patients. Our practice is to warn those over 70 years old that they may become muddled at times during the first few days, but to persevere.

Confusion may be caused by the concurrent use of morphine and psychotropic drugs. If confusional symptoms persist, a reduction in psychotropic medication should be considered (see Checklist for excessive drowsiness, p. 189).

29 Is postural hypotension a problem?

No. We advise those over 70 years old that they may experience dizziness or feel unsteady for a few days, but to persevere.

30 Constipation

This is the most troublesome unwanted effect of treatment with morphine, and with other opioids. Almost all patients become constipated unless they have an ileostomy or steatorrhoea. If not controlled, a patient may stop his medication and suffer severe pain rather than continue to be severely constipated.

Controlling constipation may be more difficult than controlling pain.

An appropriate laxative should be prescribed when morphine is started (see table opposite).

Guidelines for management of opioid-induced constipation

Ask about the patient's usual bowel habit and use of laxatives

Do rectal examination if you suspect faecal impaction or if there is diarrhoea/faecal incontinence (to exclude impaction with overflow)

Record bowel motions each day in a 'Bowel Book'

Encourage fluids generally, fruit juice, fruit and bran

Prescribe prophylactically: co-danthrusate* 1 capsule nocte *or* casanthranol 30 mg with docusate 100 mg (Peri-Colace†) 1 capsule b.i.d.

If already constipated: co-danthrusate* 2 capsules nocte *or* Peri-Colace† 2 capsules b.i.d.

Adjust every few days according to results, up to 3 capsules q.i.d.

If necessary, 'uncork' with the help of bisacodyl (Dulcolax) 10 mg suppository + glycerine suppository

If suppositories are ineffective, administer a high phosphate enema (Fleets†) followed by a soap enema if no result

If the maximum dose of co-danthrusate* *or* Peri-Colace† is ineffective, reduce by half and add an osmotic laxative ('small bowel flusher'), e.g. lactulose 30 ml b.i.d.

If co-danthrusate* *or* Peri-Colace† causes abdominal cramps divide daily dose or change to a small bowel flusher, e.g. lactulose syrup 20-40 ml daily-t.i.d.

Lactulose may be preferable in patients with a history of irritable bowel syndrome (spastic colon) or of cramps with other contact laxatives ('peristaltic stimulants'), e.g. senna

Sometimes it is appropriate to optimize a patient's existing bowel regimen, rather than change automatically to co-danthrusate* *or* Peri-Colace†

31 Sweating

Some patients complain of sweating. This can be profuse and tends to be more marked at night. It occurs more often in patients with malignant involvement of the liver, whether enlarged clinically or not. Sweating may also be troublesome in patients with a fever caused by the cancer.

Occasionally a corticosteroid (prednisolone 15–30 mg daily *or* dexamethasone 2–4 mg daily) is of benefit. Sleeping lightly clad and in a cool room may be all that one can suggest to the patient. Fortunately, most patients put up with the sweating as an acceptable price to pay for freedom from pain, especially when they understand that it has no sinister meaning.

32 What about addiction?

Psychological dependence ('addiction') does not occur in patients who are prescribed morphine for cancer pain, provided it is used within the context of total patient care.

Occasionally, a patient is admitted who appears to be addicted, demanding 'an injection' q2–3h. Typically such a patient has a long history of poor pain control, and for several weeks will have been receiving fairly regular (q4h, as required) but inadequate injections of one or more opioid analgesics.

In this situation, given time, it is usually possible to control the pain adequately, prevent the clock-watching and demanding behaviour, and eventually change progressively to an oral preparation. But even here, it cannot be said that the patient is addicted. He is not demanding the opioid in order to experience its psychological effect but to be relieved from pain for at least an hour or two.

Physical dependence develops in most patients who have taken opioids regularly for more than 3–4 weeks. This is not a problem for most dying patients as they will continue on regular morphine until they die.

Some patients live for much longer than expected. If their pain disappears, morphine can be sequentially decreased and possibly stopped altogether. Guidelines are as follows

■ If a patient — usually an outpatient — has been entirely pain free for 4–8 weeks, on a regular unchanged dose of morphine, and is in general relatively well, reduce the dose by a convenient amount (this will vary from 20–50%)

■ If the pain recurs, increase the dose back to the original level

■ If the pain does not return and the patient feels well, decrease the dose again after 7–10 days

■ Do *not* lengthen the intervals between doses

33 Do patients die of morphine-induced respiratory depression?

No. This is because pain antagonizes the central depressant effects of morphine. When morphine is used in the way described in this guide, significant respiratory depression is rarely seen. Should it occur

- Reduce the dose of morphine if the patient is pain-free

- Consider alternative drug and non-drug treatments

- Consider using a cerebral stimulant (*rarely indicated*)

'Blunderbus' or 'shotgun' therapy is, however, always dangerous. We have seen patients whose death was possibly precipitated by an excessive initial dose of morphine.

Overdosage may occur if the dose of morphine is increased automatically on 'chart rounds', without careful bedside reassessment.

34   Are there any circumstances in which treatment with morphine has to be abandoned?

On rare occasions, yes. Details are shown in the table overleaf.

More Questions About Morphine

35 Why do some people need more morphine than others?

There are many reasons why this is so. They include

- Difference in pain intensity

- Use or non-use of adjuvant drugs and non-drug measures

- Pharmacokinetic differences
  - absorption
  - 'first pass' hepatic metabolism
  - plasma half-life
  - renal function

- Fundamental differences in patient's pain tolerance threshold (relates to central nervous system endorphin stores)

- Acquired differences in patient's pain tolerance threshold (relates mainly to mood and morale)

- Previously induced tolerance
  - needless increases in dose
  - initial use of morphine by injection in excessive amounts

Morphine intolerance

Type	Effects	Initial action	Comment
Gastric stasis	Epigastric fullness, flatulence, anorexia, persistent nausea	Antiflatulent antacid 10 ml q4h and metoclopramide 10–20 mg q4h	If persists, change to chemically distinct opioid, e.g. phenazocine*, levorphanol, methadone
Psychotomimetic	Notably dysphoria and hallucinations	Haloperidol 3–5mg nocte	
Vestibular stimulation	Incapacitating movement-induced nausea and vomiting	Cyclizine 50–100 mg q4h *or* meclozine† 25 mg q8–12h	Rare. Try alternative opioid or methotrimeprazine
Histamine release (a) bronchial	Bronchoconstriction →dyspnoea	Antihistamine IV/IM (e.g. chlorpheniramine 5–10 mg) and bronchodilator	Very rare. Change to chemically distinct opioid immediately
(b) cutaneous	Pruritus	Oral antihistamine (e.g. chlorpheniramine 4 mg b.-t.i.d.)	If the intolerance does not settle after a few days or reappears when the antihistamine is stopped, prescribe alternative opioid

- Previous inadequate use of strong opioids, especially 'as required' injections for continuous pain

- Previous use of strong opioids

- Duration of treatment (overall tendency for the dose to increase as the disease progresses)

- Adequacy of control of other distressing symptoms

36 Is oral morphine really effective?

Yes. Morphine sulphate/hydrochloride has been used in doses q4h ranging from as little as 5 mg *up to 1200 mg*. Published data show that for aqueous morphine

- The median maximum dose is 15–20 mg

- Few patients ever need more than 200 mg

- Patients poorly controlled on 100 mg may obtain benefit at higher doses

Controlled trials have shown that SR tablets are equally efficacious. This means that, for SR morphine, the median maximum dose is likely to be about 60 mg b.i.d. and few patients will need more than 600 mg b.i.d.

It is only rarely necessary to prescribe morphine by injection because oral morphine is not working.

37 Is it necessary to give more morphine by mouth than by injection?

Yes. As a general rule, the dose of morphine sulphate should be doubled when converting to the oral route. If this proves inadequate increase to 3 times the injected dose.

The much-quoted 6-fold conversion ratio is incorrect. It relates to a single-dose study: it does not hold for regular administration. Giving 6 times as much morphine by mouth as by injection will cause oversedation and respiratory depression.

38 Wouldn't injections be better?

No. Injections are *not* better, and can be uncomfortable. Injections also tend to tie the patient unnecessarily to a second person, usually a nurse, because usually someone else is needed to administer the medication.

39 In what situations do injections become necessary?

Main	Subsidiary
Intractable vomiting	Psychological aversion to oral
Inability to swallow	medication
Coma	Poor alimentary absorption (rare)

If regular injections become necessary, a *continuous SC infusion of morphine* is preferable to repeated SC/IM doses. A range of portable syringe drivers are available. Graseby Medical, Braun and Pharmacia are all widely used.

When changing to injections, the dose of morphine should be halved.

In the UK, diamorphine* (diacetylmorphine, heroin) is commonly used as the *parenteral* strong opioid of choice. When converting from oral morphine to parenteral diamorphine* the dose of oral morphine sulphate should be *divided by 3* to determine the dose of diamorphine hydrochloride*.

In the USA, hydromorphone† is commonly used for parenteral administration. The dose of oral morphine should be *divided by 6* to determine the dose of hydromorphone†.

40 Once on injections, is it possible to change successfully to the oral route?

Once vomiting has been controlled with parenteral antiemetics, it is often possible to convert to oral medication (both analgesic and antiemetic).

It may be wise, however, to convert to the oral route in stages. For example, the antiemetic can be changed first, followed the next day by the 0600 h and 1000 h dose of morphine. Finally, the other doses can be changed. The 'run-in' period with the other medication will show whether a complete change to oral medication is feasible. A progressive conversion is also wise if a patient cannot believe that oral medication will be effective.

41   When close to death and the patient becomes unconscious, should the morphine be discontinued?

No. Mainly for two reasons

■   Unconscious patients in pain tend to become restless

■   Physical dependence develops after several weeks of oral morphine therapy. If the morphine is stopped abruptly, the patient will become restless, sweaty, and might develop faecal incontinence secondary to rebound hyperperistalsis

It does, however, take only a quarter of the analgesic dose to prevent opioid withdrawal symptoms and signs.

42   Can morphine be given by suppository?

Yes. Suppositories of morphine sulphate are availabe in a range of strengths from 10–60 mg* (5–30 mg†). They can also be made by any helpful pharmacist. The oral to rectal potency ratio is 1:1. In other words, the same amount is needed PR as PO to control pain. Suppositories are a useful alternative to injections, particularly in the home.

If administration q4h proves difficult, it is possible to give SR morphine tablets q12h PR. Pharmacokinetic studies have demonstrated that they are equally well absorbed by this route.

In the USA, oxymorphone† is available as a 10 mg suppository. Oxymorphone* is twice as potent as morphine by this route, i.e. each 10 mg suppository is equivalent to 20 mg of morphine.

43   What's so special about 'q4h'?

Extensive clinical experience has shown that increasing the dose of aqueous morphine to provide relief for 4 h achieves the optimum balance between relief, practical convenience, and unwanted effects.

Giving more at less frequent intervals will provide comfort for a longer period but only at the price of more troublesome unwanted effects, particularly drowsiness.

Giving less at more frequent intervals simply makes the regular taking of morphine more tedious for the patient, especially at night. Compliance is then reduced and increased pain is the end result.

The general rule is: *give aqueous morphine regularly q4h.*

44 For aqueous morphine, are there any exceptions to the q4h rule?

Regular aqueous morphine q4h is indicated for continuous pain, *not* for occasional pain. The following are also circumstances in which it may be desirable to prescribe aqueous morphine *less* than q4h.

- The very old (90 +)
  - □ initially
  - □ indefinitely

- Patients with night pain only

- Patients with evening and night pain only

- Patients in renal failure

45 Is it ever necessary to give morphine more often than q4h?

Yes. Very occasionally a patient appears to metabolize morphine exceptionally fast. Increasing the dose in an attempt to prolong relief from 3 h to 4 h does little except increase unwanted effects.

46 How can I tell if administration q3h is indicated?

The following questions will help you decide

'Is the pain completely absent from one dose of medicine to the next?' If the answer is 'No', then ask: 'Does the pain completely go, but come back before your next medicine is due, or does the medicine just ease the pain, but never make you pain-free?'

If it just eases, a morphine increment is clearly required. If it goes and returns, the patient *may* be a fast metabolizer. The correct course is to increase the morphine by one or two increments and monitor both relief and unwanted effects. If there is *minimal* improvement in pain relief but a considerable increase in unwanted effects (drowsiness, vomiting), revert to the former smaller dose and take it q3h.

q3h is, however, more inconvenient to the patient and his family than q4h. Therefore, the first step is always to increase the dose of morphine sulphate rather than immediately reducing the interval between doses.

It is most unusual to need to give morphine q3h.

The above advice is given on the assumption that the physician is treating a morphine responsive pain and that appropriate non-drug measures are being employed. As emphasized elsewhere, attempts to obliterate morphine non-responsive and activity-precipitated pains with morphine usually result in serious unwanted effects.

47 Should patients be awakened to take a dose in the middle of the night?

Theoretically: yes. In practice: often no. In the following circumstances, a dose in the middle of the night is advisable.

■ Some patients already taking analgesics during the night have become established in a routine. It may not be wise to break this routine, at least immediately

■ The patient wakes regularly to micturate between 0100 h and 0300 h. Here it is unnecessary to attempt all-night analgesic cover. The patient can take a dose when he wakes to micturate

■ Attempts to achieve all night relief have failed, and the patient continues to wake in pain in the second half of the night (0300–0600 h)

48 Can a dose in the middle of the night be avoided in other circumstances?

Yes. We regard it as the norm for the patient to sleep through the night without a dose at 0200 h. This has been achieved by modifying the 'q4h' regimen to:

q4h during the day (0600, 1000, 1400, 1800 h) and *a double dose at bedtime* (2200 h).

The greater unwanted effect liability of morphine when given in a larger dose q4h is turned to good effect: the patient sleeps more soundly.

49   Is a double dose more dangerous?

In the very frail and/or elderly, particularly if there is a risk that
they might wake in the night disoriented or feeling 'drugged', it is
wise to start with a 50% higher dose at bedtime, rather than a
double dose. In most patients, however, a double dose of
morphine at bedtime is perfectly safe.

50   What about the Brompton Cocktail?

This traditional British mixture of morphine sulphate and cocaine
in a vehicle of syrup, alcohol and chloroform water offers no
advantages over aqueous morphine. On the other hand, it causes
more unwanted effects. It is more nauseating (due to the syrup
content) and may cause a burning sensation in the throat (due to
the alcohol). If a patient finds the plain morphine solution
unacceptably bitter, he should be advised to add milk, fruit juice,
or other flavouring at the time of administration. Alternatively, a
proprietary preparation of morphine sulphate or hydrochloride
could be prescribed as these include a masking taste.

51   Is diamorphine* (heroin) better than morphine?

By mouth, morphine and diamorphine* (diacetylmorphine,
heroin) have similar actions and unwanted effects but, because it
is more completely absorbed, oral diamorphine* is about 1.5
times more potent than oral morphine. It is, however, no more
efficacious. By the time diamorphine* reaches the brain it has
been deacetylated, that is, metabolized to morphine.
Diamorphine* is, in fact, a pro-drug of morphine.

52   What about driving?

Most patients receiving morphine are not well enough to drive,
and have no wish to do so. Some are much stronger and are
continuing to work. For patients who wish to drive we give the
following advice:

The medicines you are taking do *not* necessarily disqualify you
from driving. The speed of your reactions and general alertness
may, however, be affected by your medication.

It is important that you take the following precautions,
particularly if you have not driven for some weeks because of ill
health

- Do not drive in the dark or when conditions are bad

- Do not drink alcohol, however little, during the day

- Check your fitness to drive in the following way
  - □ choose a quiet time of the day, when the light is good
  - □ choose an area where there are a number of quiet roads
  - □ take a companion (husband, wife, friend)
  - □ drive for 10–15 minutes on quiet roads
  - □ if both you and your companion are happy with your attentiveness, reactions and general ability, then it is all right to drive for short distances

- Do not exhaust yourself by long journeys

Doctors have an ethical and legal responsibility to advise patients if a disability is likely to make them a danger when driving. In many states and countries, there is an obligation on the driver to report any such disability to the licensing authority, unless relatively short-term (e.g. less than 3 months). The patient can, however, fulfil his obligation only if his doctor advises him appropriately.

In some districts of the USA, there are driving evaluation centres. An assessment at one of these will provide an objective assessment of a person's capability to drive.

53 If morphine is prescribed more than a few weeks before a patient's death, what happens when tolerance develops?

When morphine is used regularly, prophylactically in individually optimized doses, and within the context of 'total patient care', tolerance is not a practical problem. Many patients continue on an unchanged dose for weeks or months. In some, it is possible to reduce the dose after several weeks without any breakthrough pain. Rapid escalation of dose is not necessary when morphine is used properly.

54 Don't patients die quickly once morphine has been prescribed?

Many patients prescribed morphine are near to death and remain near to death. These will die quickly. On the other hand, in our experience, one-third of patients survive more than 4 weeks; 10% for more than 3 months.

Whether the patient dies in a short time depends at what stage morphine therapy is started. Circumstantial evidence suggests that many patients survive for a longer period because they are able to rest, sleep, eat more, and take a renewed interest in life.

On the other hand, giving morphine to an exhausted cachectic patient (from long unrelieved pain and insomnia), especially if elderly, may lead to pneumonia as a result of somnolence and cough suppression. When used in the way described in this guide, however, the risk is very small.

55 If patients have morphine at home, won't it get stolen?

We know of no patient whose morphine was stolen by intruders. There have been rare reports of misappropriation by a relative or a friend.

56 Won't patients use their morphine to commit suicide?

We know of no example of self-poisoning by a cancer patient in which the agent used was a solution of morphine sulphate. The incidence of suicide in cancer patients is, in any case, not above that of the general population.

57 Isn't the use of morphine tantamount to prescribing a 'living death'?

Many doctors and nurses have a markedly negative attitude towards the medicinal use of morphine. As one doctor wrote:

> 'What about the inoperable cancer patient who may not die for months or a year, and yet who is suffering agonies from chronic pain?... Is a doctor then justified in prescribing such drugs when he knows full well he will be sentencing his patient to a kind of living death?'

And although they might not express it so succinctly, many doctors still share the view of the physician who said:

> 'I try to postpone giving morphia until the very end and am best pleased if the first dose of morphia is also the last.'

These views stem from ignorance about and misunderstanding of the correct use of morphine in cancer patients with pain. Indeed, the patients who are truly sentenced to 'a kind of living death' are the ones who are *not* prescribed an adequate analgesic regimen. One such man had been bedridden because of pain for 2 months. His wife then found him crawling around the living room on his hands and knees searching for his gun which she had hidden for fear he would shoot himself. The subsequent correct use of morphine enabled this patient to live a far more normal life than would otherwise have been possible. The same is true for many others, as a visit to any good hospice will demonstrate.

58   Is oral morphine the panacea for cancer pain?

Definitely not! Oral morphine sulphate is a useful treatment modality without which life would be extremely uncomfortable for many patients with advanced cancer. It must be used correctly with an awareness of its limitations and of the need for regular close supervision.

59   What are the more important non-drug treatments?

■   Psychological support of the patient and family

■   Modification of pattern of living (for pains precipitated or exacerbated by activity)

■   Radiation therapy (principally for bone pain)

■   Nerve blocks (principally for intractable nerve compression pains)

There are, of course, many other non-drug treatments — too many to list here.

60   When treating the cancer patient in pain, what else must I bear in mind?

The International Association for the Study of Pain defines pain as *an unpleasant sensory and emotional experience* associated with actual or potential tissue damage, or described in terms of such damage.

As pain is a somatopsychic experience, its intensity is modified by a person's emotional reaction to the physical component.

Those caring for the patient with cancer must be aware of all the interacting factors which influence the patient's perception of his discomfort. The following diagram indicates some of the many non-physical influences that modify a patient's perception of pain.

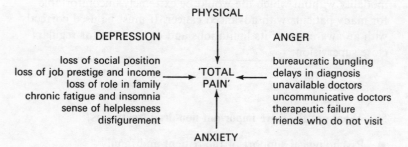

Factors influencing pain sensitivity

other symptoms
side effects of treatment

PHYSICAL

DEPRESSION   ANGER

loss of social position   bureaucratic bungling
loss of job prestige and income   → 'TOTAL ← delays in diagnosis
loss of role in family   PAIN'   unavailable doctors
chronic fatigue and insomnia   uncommunicative doctors
sense of helplessness   therapeutic failure
disfigurement   friends who do not visit

ANXIETY

fear of hospital or nursing home
fear of pain
worry about family and finances
fear of death
spiritual unrest, uncertainty about future

If you are not prepared to attempt to treat all the many factors influencing the perception of pain, it would perhaps be wise not to prescribe morphine, but to ask a colleague who is more willing, and possibly more able, to look after your patient.

'As the doctor-patient relationship improved, many doctors found they could reduce the drugs. As the true diagnosis of the patient's pain became clear and the patient was helped to deal with the pain of dying, there was less need for sedatives, tranquillizers, and analgesics.'

(Harte)

'No-one who hasn't time for chat knows anything about terminal care, however brilliant a clinical pharmacologist he may be.'

(Smithers)

Other Important Uses of Morphine

61 How is morphine used to relieve dyspnoea?

Patients with dyspnoea due to irreversible malignant chest disease often benefit from the prescription of oral morphine.

The use of morphine is aimed at reducing the *sensation* of breathlessness, and implies that:

- Reversible factors, e.g. heart failure and bronchospasm, have been treated

- General guidance about coping with dyspnoea has been given

- An anxiolytic has been prescribed, e.g. diazepam 5-10 mg nocte

If a resting respiratory rate of 30/per min, rising to 40/min or more on mild exertion, distresses and frightens the patient, it should be treated. As with pain relief, aqueous morphine should be given q4h to patients with dyspnoea. (See section 44 for exceptions to this rule.)

Much of the benefit from morphine relates to a reduction in a futile respiratory 'overdrive' that is commonly seen in patients with diffuse pulmonary malignant disease. This is possibly caused by the respiratory stimulant effect of atelectasis.

62 What is the right dose of morphine for dyspnoea?

The dose of morphine to reduce dyspnoea tends to be smaller than that used to relieve pain

- Start with a test dose of 5 mg

- Continue with 5 mg q4h, 5–10 mg nocte

- If there is no benefit at all and no unwanted effects, increase next day to 10 mg q4h, 15–20 mg nocte

- If there is some benefit but the resting respiratory rate remains > 24/min, increase the dose after 2–3 days and review

- Consider further adjustment to morphine 15–20 mg q4h after 2–3 more days

■ If a patient is already receiving morphine for pain control, the dose of morphine should be increased by 50% on a trial basis

At each stage, benefits must be weighed against unwanted effects. The aim is a more relaxed patient who is not cyanosed and is mentally clear-headed.

63 Is oral morphine of value in other forms of terminal illness?

Yes. There are at least two other situations in which morphine should be considered:

■ To ease the aches and discomforts of the patient who is slowly dying and bedbound
Small daytime doses, i.e. 5 mg q4h and a larger bedtime dose, i.e. 10–15 mg, if the nights are disturbed by pain-linked insomnia, may make a considerable difference to the bodily and mental comfort of the dying.

■ As a cough sedative, and/or night sedative in patients with motor neurone disease (amyotrophic lateral sclerosis)

Most patients with this disorder develop a pseudobulbar palsy, i.e., progressive impairment of the lower cranial nerves. This results in progressive dysphonia and dysphagia. Associated with the dysphagia is a tendency to choke unpredictably when eating or drinking, and at night, as a result of aspiration of saliva. The resulting terror and anticipatory fear is a major problem in the management of terminal motor neurone disease.

While dietary advice and explanation may help, a cough sedative is generally necessary to prevent or minimize the bouts of choking. Depending on the circumstances, we start on either oral morphine sulphate 3–5 mg nocte or b.i.d. and go on to titrate dose and frequency in the light of the initial response. Most patients need only 5 mg t.i.d. before meals with perhaps a larger bedtime dose. A few take it q4h.

11 PSYCHOSOCIAL ISSUES

Biopsychosocial care
Communication
Adjusting to a poor
   prognosis

Hope
Care of the relatives
Appropriate treatment
Teamwork

Biopsychosocial Care

Care of the dying extends far beyond pain relief and the alleviation
of other symptoms — important though these are. It includes

■ Supporting the patient emotionally as he adjusts to his
decreasing physical ability and as he mourns in anticipation the
loss of his family, his friends and all that is familiar

■ Supporting the family as they adjust to the fact that one of
them is dying

Although emotionally demanding for doctor and nurse, it is
potentially one of the most rewarding of their responsibilities.

Fear

All of us fear death; it is part of the survival instinct. We feel
uneasy in life-threatening situations. We also feel uneasy in the
presence of death. There is therefore a natural tendency to
withdraw from those who are dying.

Frequently the dying patient is not involved in discussions about
his illness in the same way as other patients. This causes
resentment, and symptoms tend to multiply or worsen.

On the other hand, if the dying patient is treated as a person and
not as someone to be feared and avoided, it is usually possible to
maintain a patient's self-respect and morale. This means
employing the common courtesies

■ Greet the patient by name and shake hands

- If you have not met the patient before, introduce yourself; give your name and the reason for the visit

- Whenever possible sit down. This is imperative when discussing life-threatening issues

- Listen to what the patient has to say

- Whenever possible, involve him in the making of decisions about treatment and continuing care

Many patients have fears relating to

- Separation from family, home or job

- The completion of unfinished tasks

- The consequences for dependents

- Losing control of physical and mental faculties

- Being dependent on others

- Being 'useless' or 'no good to anybody'

- 'Being a nuisance'

- Mutilation or pain

- An undignified or 'messy' death

- Dying alone

Few patients talk to a doctor about their fears, particularly the more diffuse, less well defined fear of death. This may be because doctors lack time. Many doctors convey the impression of being unwilling to communicate at this level. Given an unhurried atmosphere and the doctor's willingness to discuss such matters, many dying patients appreciate the opportunity to talk.

Spiritual Care

It is important to discover what the patient's spiritual needs are. Whether apparent or not, most patients are in need of spiritual help and are seeking answers to questions such as

- *The meaning of life* What is the meaning of life in a time of serious illness?

- *Value systems* What value is there in money, material possessions, and social position?

- *Meaning of suffering and pain* Why do I have to suffer? Why do I have to have pain?

- *Guilt feelings* I have done many wrong things; how can they be corrected? How can I be forgiven?

- *Quest after God* Is there a God? Why does God allow me to suffer like this?

- *Life after death* Is there life after death? How can I believe in life after death?

Only a minority of patients discuss the spiritual aspects of life and death with their doctor. The majority do so with another team member, with relatives or close friends.

- It is important to recognize that the dying do consider such issues and be able to respond sympathetically if a patient chooses to raise them

- Patients are very perceptive, they are unlikely to embarrass a doctor if they sense that communication at this level will cause discomfort

- A doctor's prime responsibility is to help maintain an environment which is supportive of the patient. This requires control of symptoms so that the patient is able to consider these issues

- When appropriate, the doctor should alert the chaplain, priest, or rabbi to the fact that: 'Mr X is seriously ill and may appreciate a visit'

Regard for the patient as an individual does not allow the imposition of one's own faith, or lack of it, on him.

Many patients are comforted by the discovery that their doctor has a religious faith.

Communication

It is not a matter of 'to communicate or not to communicate' but a question of good versus bad communication. The basic message a patient wants to hear at a time of increasing uncertainty is:

'No matter what happens to you, I am going to do all I can to help you.'

'You may have cancer/you may be dying, but you are still important to me.'

Only part of this can be said in words:

'We will continue to take good care of you.'
'I will see you regularly.'
'One of us will always be available.'
'We will deal with any problems that arise.'
'We can relieve your pain and can control most other symptoms.'

Essentially this fundamental message of support and companionship is conveyed to the patient by means of non-verbal and indirect verbal communication. This probably accounts for 80% of all communication between doctor and patient.

Practical Points

- Employ common courtesies
- Sit down if possible
- Make eye to eye contact
- Visit regularly

Begin conversation with a positive comment:

'Hullo, Mrs Smith, it's good to see you.'

Avoid greetings that may evoke a negative response:

'Good morning, Mrs Smith, how are you?'
'Good morning, Mrs Smith, did you sleep well last night?'

Attention to detail: ask questions about known specific symptoms. Also ask about:
- sleep
- general comfort
- diet
- mouth
- bowels
- micturition

Warning: If another doctor has already visited the patient that day, try to avoid repetitive enquiry. Instead, chat as friend to friend. 'Clinical sensitivity' is needed to find right balance.

- examine — check pulse and respiration
  - legs — for sore heels; dry itchy skin; oedema
  - back — at least once a week to check sacral skin
  - abdomen — if affected by disease or if doubt about status of bowels
  - chest — if affected by disease or if complaint of dyspnoea or cough
  - breasts — at least once a week if ulcerated or in danger of ulcerating
  - mouth — for dryness; coating; Candidiasis
- Physical contact — touching, whether holding the patient's hand or feeling his pulse, is an important non-verbal form of reassurance and comfort.

Verbal Communication

Initially, when the patient's condition is diagnosed, he needs to be told what is wrong with him, in words that he can understand, and what medical science has to offer him.

For most people, cancer is an emotive word and to answer a direct question with, 'Yes, I'm afraid you have cancer', is unwise unless qualified. If used, it is important to discover what the patient understands by cancer. If it means a painful and distressing death, he needs to be reassured that treatments are available to relieve pain and other symptoms should they develop.

In practice it is seldom a question of 'to tell or not to tell', but more a matter of 'when and how to tell'.

A patient's questions or statements often open the way:

'And what's the next step, doctor?'
'When will I be able to go home?'
'How long do you reckon this will go on, doctor?'
'I'm not getting any better, am I?'
'I know I'm going to die.'
'I know what I've got.'
'I've got cancer, haven't I, doctor?'

Such remarks usually mean that the patient wants more information, that he is ready to accept more of the truth even if it is unpalatable.

If at a certain stage, a patient indicates by his manner and talk that he does not wish to regard his illness as fatal, it is wrong to force the truth upon him. Few patients adopt such a stance permanently.

Cardinal Principles in Communication

■ Explain the reasons for the symptoms

■ Generally, patients who want to know more about their condition will ask, if the way is opened to them

■ A formal ward round with entourage is not the best milieu. Visit the patient alone on another occasion, sit down to show that you have time, and gradually lead conversation towards the illness. This is facilitated by appropriate leading questions:

'What things have been running through your mind as to the possible cause of your symptoms?'
'This illness has been going on for rather a long time, how do you see things working out?'
'How do you think you are getting on?'
'Are you worried about yourself?'
'How are t[family coping with you still being ill?'

■ Generally, patients who do not want to know will not ask

■ Do not compromise your relationship with the patient by making unwise (and unethical) promises to the relatives about non-disclosure of information to the patient

■ Truth has a broad spectrum with gentleness at one end and harshness at the other. Patients always prefer gentle truth. As far as possible soften the *initial* impact of emotionally negative words:

Not 'You have got cancer'
But 'Tests indicate that it is a form of cancer'

Not 'You have got three months to live'
But 'Time is probably limited'

Euphemism is legitimate if used to express truth gently; it is wrong if used to deceive

■ Express bad news by using words with positive rather than negative overtones:

Not 'You have got *weaker*'
But 'At the moment, energy is limited'

Not 'Things are getting *worse*'
But 'Things don't seem to be so good this week'

■ The doctor-patient relationship is founded on trust. It is fostered by honesty but poisoned by deceit

■ The doctor's responsibility is to nudge the patient in the direction of reality but never to force him

■ 'The aim is to make dying a little easier, not to apply the dogma of always divulging the truth' (Hinton)

Adjusting to a Poor Prognosis

People cope with crises in life by using a variety of defence or coping mechanisms.

These enable the person to continue to function without excessive anxiety, depression or anger, and provide a 'breathing space' during which the person can adapt to the new situation.

Common defence mechanisms

Denial	Regression
Compensation	Intellectualization
Displacement	Religious faith
Projection	Fatalism
Dependency	Stoicism

In the dying, the commonest defence mechanism is probably *denial*. It takes a variety of forms but basically implies an ability to obliterate or minimize reality by ignoring it. It may however be associated with physiological and non-verbal evidence of anxiety. With time, most patients make less use of denial.

Compensation is an extreme form of denial in which the patient overcompensates for the limitations imposed by the illness, and the associated fears, by being excessively active and joyful.

None of these mechanisms is in itself maladaptive though the persistent use of some may become so. A defence mechanism is maladaptive if its continued use causes additional suffering to the patient. It is important to recognize maladaption and seek additional psychotherapeutic help if it persists.

Adjustments

As denial gives way to other methods of coping there may be episodes of

- Anger
- Anxiety
- Depression

Those around the patient need to recognize these as part of the process of adjustment. Only then can anger and frustration in the care givers (potentially damaging to all concerned) be avoided or contained.

Honesty and sensitivity assist the patient in his progress through a series of adjustments to a new psychological equilibrium.

- Adjustment to a poor prognosis takes time
- Different coping mechanisms are employed by different patients
- Any one patient may utilize several mechanisms simultaneously or at different stages during the period of adjustment
- Patients cope less well with naked truth at first. The initial blow may be softened by stressing what medical science has to offer, erring on the side of optimism

Most patients adapt to the fact that they have a limited prognosis.

'*Accept and fight*' describes the approach of many. Acceptance is different from resignation. Acceptance brings something positive to the patient. Resignation is essentially negative and casts a shadow across the final phase of the patient's illness.

'*Total ambivalence*' describes the psychological stance adopted by some patients. 'I wish it could all be over soon' — but eager to eat, presumably to maintain strength and ward off death. Acceptance is at an intellectual level only.

'*Total surrender*' is also seen. Here the patient says 'I am ready to die' when it is biologically premature. It tends to result in a prolonged period of inactivity because the patient is unable to harness his limited stamina to maximum advantage. It is commonly not possible to change this pattern of behaviour. It is therefore necessary to support the patient within the constraints of his chosen attitude.

'*Reject and rage*' is perhaps the most maladaptive attitude, and the most distressing for the family and those caring for the patient. Fortunately, it occurs infrequently. The fortitude of the majority of dying patients encourages the doctor and provides the emotional resources for dealing with a seemingly totally negative situation.

There is no one right way of adjusting to a poor prognosis. The doctor's task is to help the patient do his best given that particular patient's background — genetic, familial, cultural and spiritual.

Hope

'An expectation greater than zero of achieving a goal'.

Hope tends to diminish when

- The patient is mentally isolated by a 'conspiracy of silence'
- It is implied 'there is nothing more that can be done'
- Pain and other symptoms remain unrelieved or even ignored
- The patient feels alone or unsupported

'Never destroy hope' is frequently used as a reason for not informing a patient of the seriousness of his situation. Yet glib, false optimism is a potent destroyer of hope.

Gentle, sympathetic and gradual communication of the truth within the context of continued support and encouragement does much to restore and maintain hope.

Communication of painful truth does not equal destruction of hope. Hope of recovery is often replaced by an alternative hope

- The hope of good symptom control
- The hope of a peaceful death
- The hope that one's life has been worthwhile
- The hope of immortality in some form
- The hope that one's loved ones will cope on their own

Care of the Relatives

The care of the family is an integral part of the care of the dying.

A contented family increases the likelihood of a contented patient.

Relative-doctor communication generally needs to be *initiated* and *maintained* by the doctor. It is easy to neglect relatives because of their reluctance to bother the doctor.

Telling the Relatives

There is much to be said for joint interviews, both at the time of diagnosis and later — patient, relative, doctor and nurse. The nurse is then better qualified to clarify the doctor's statements and to respond to ongoing concerns.

The doctor should also make an opportunity to see both the patient and the close family apart from each other. Further separate or joint interviews can then be arranged as necessary.

As with the patient, it is generally not necessary or wise to tell the family the whole truth (as you see it) at one time. The relatives also need to adjust to the implications of the illness.

For the family and patient to be too far 'out of step' in relation to knowledge about the diagnosis and the prognosis can create a barrier between them.

■ A common initial reaction is 'You won't tell him, will you, doctor?' or 'We'd prefer you not to tell him, doctor'. This should be seen as the initial shock reaction and not used as an excuse for saying nothing to the patient

■ Generally, such reactions are not based on compassion but reflect anxiety in the relatives and stem from their own instinctive fear of death

■ If the family and patient are to be mutually supportive it is necessary to help the relatives move forward from this initial reaction to a position of greater openness and trust

■ The family *cannot* forbid the doctor from discussion of diagnosis and prognosis with the patient.

Involvement in Hospital Care

Admission to hospital is often seen as a defeat by the family.

It is necessary to emphasize that you are surprised that they had managed to cope for so long and that now, with the need for day and night care, it is impossible for one (or two) people to continue alone without a break.

■ Encourage frequent visits if practical, and emphasize how important you regard the presence of relatives and close friends

■ Help to reduce the relative's separation anxiety by encouraging them to help in the care of the patient - adjusting pillows, refilling a water jug, helping with a blanket bath, assisting at meals if necessary

■ Some relatives need to be taught how to visit, to behave as they would at home, e.g. sit and read a book or newspaper, knit, watch the television together. Emphasize that they don't have to keep up a tiring patter of conversation

■ Arrange overnight accommodation when necessary

Planning for Discharge

A proportion of patients with terminal cancer improve following admission as a result of the control of pain and other symptoms. They become physically independent again and no longer need to be in hospital.

Many relatives have fears about what will happen should the patient be discharged. A trial day out or weekend at home does much to allay their fears (or confirms that discharge is after all impractical).

■ Talk with the relatives (as well as the patient) *before* and *after* trial periods at home and plan on the basis of comments by both family and patient

■ Give clear advice about whom to call in the event of a crisis

The Right Balance

Patients are sometimes overprotected by their family. They are prevented from driving and from visiting the pub or betting shop, even though still capable of doing so.

It is necessary in these cases to help the relatives to accept the patient's need (and right) to maintain the maximum possible degree of independence.

An explanation that a sudden dramatic deterioration is unlikely will help ease the family's apprehension, as will clear guidance on what to do in an emergency.

Explanation of Treatment

Terminally, it is advisable to tell the relatives that, because the patient is less well, his medicine may need to be given *regularly* by injection to prevent a resurgence of pain.

When pneumonia supervenes, it is sometimes advisable to explain that you are not going to use antibiotics, but plan to continue treating symptomatically.

After the Patient's Death

As bereavement has both a morbidity and a mortality, terminal care does not end when the patient dies.

Many relatives have false feelings of guilt:

'If only I'd done this!'

'Do you think if he'd gone to the hospital sooner, etc?'

Opportunity should be given for such feelings to be aired and questions to be raised.

Appropriate Treatment

In terminal illness the primary aim is no longer to preserve life but to make the life that remains as comfortable and as meaningful as possible.

What may be appropriate treatment in an acutely ill patient may be inappropriate in the dying.

Cardiac resuscitation, artificial respiration, IV infusions, nasogastric tubes, and antibiotics are primarily supportive measures for use in acute or acute-on-chronic illnesses to assist a patient through the initial period towards recovery of health. To use such measures in the terminally ill, with no expectancy of a return to health, is generally inappropriate and is therefore bad medicine.

Such measures can be ethically used only if they are clearly contributing to the immediate comfort of the patient.

It is not a question of 'to treat or not to treat?' but, rather, a matter of what is appropriate treatment from a biological point of view in a particular patient. Some patients suffer as much from inappropriate treatment as they do from the underlying illness

Medical treatment should be seen as a continuum ranging from cure to palliative care. When cure is no longer possible control should be considered; when control is no longer possible, the emphasis moves to palliative care.

Many types of treatment span the entire spectrum, for example, radiotherapy and also, to a lesser extent, chemotherapy and surgery. It is important not to put a particular type of treatment into a rigid category but to keep the therapeutic aim clearly in mind when employing treatment of any kind.

■ A doctor is not bound legally, morally or ethically to preserve life 'at all costs', rather life should be sustained when from a biological point of view it is sustainable

■ Priorities change when a patient is clearly dying

■ There is no obligation to employ treatments if their use can best be described as prolonging the process of dying

■ A doctor has no right to prescribe a lingering death

Teamwork

No one individual is able to provide for all the physical, mental and spiritual needs of a dying person; many people will be involved.

As death approaches, continuity of management is increasingly important, and good communication within the caring team is vital.

The doctor's involvement will vary, though matters will be greatly helped by a continued close interest, even if the situation seems straightforward. The doctor's presence is a source of encouragement to the patient and his family, and also to the nurses and other staff involved.

The basic aim is to help the person who is dying do his best given his personality, family, cultural background, physical symptoms and philosophy of life and death.

Terminal illness should not be regarded simply as an intrusion into life. It is part of life and, rightly handled, can be a time of increasing maturity and deepening spiritual insight for all concerned.

APPENDIX

Selected Drug Doses in Terminal Cancer

[Based mainly on experience at Sir Michael Sobell House, Oxford]

Drug	Modal[1] dose	Range[2]
Analgesics		
aspirin	600 mg q4h	600–1000 mg q6h
paracetamol/ acetaminophen	1 g q4h	1 g q8h–1 g q4h
flurbiprofen	100 mg q12h	50 mg q12h–100 mg q8h
naproxen diflunisal }	500 mg q12h	250–500 mg q12h
codeine (for diarrhoea)		30 mg q12h–120 mg q4h
co-proxamol* (tabs)	2 q4h	2 q6h–3 q4h
morphine (aqueous)		5 mg q6h–600 mg q4h
morphine (slow-release)		10 mg nocte–600 mg q12h
phenazocine*		2.5 mg q6h–20 mg q4h
buprenorphine		0.2 mg q8h–1 mg q6h
Antiemetics		
haloperidol	1.5 mg nocte	1.5–20 mg nocte
fluphenazine	1 mg b.i.d.	0.5 mg b.i.d.–2 mg t.i.d.
metoclopramide domperidone* }	10 mg q4h	10 mg q8h–20 mg q4h
cyclizine	50 mg b.i.d.	50 mg b.i.d.–100 mg t.i.d.
meclozine†	25 mg b.i.d.	25 mg b.i.d.–t.i.d.

Drug	Modal[1] dose	Range[2]
Laxatives		
senna	15 mg b.i.d.	7.5–75 mg a day
co-danthrusate* (caps)	2 b.i.d.	1 nocte–3 q.i.d.
Peri-Colace† (caps)	2 t.i.d.	1 nocte–3 q.i.d.
docusate	200 mg b.i.d.	200 mg daily–300 mg b.i.d.
lactulose (syrup)	30 ml q12h	10 ml daily–40 ml q8h
magnesium sulphate (crystals)	5 ml daily	2.5 ml daily–15 ml b.i.d.
Corticosteroids		
prednisolone	15 mg daily	10 mg daily–20 mg t.i.d.
dexamethasone	4 mg daily	2 mg daily–6 mg q4h
fludrocortisone	0.1 mg daily	0.05–0.3 mg daily
Psychotropic drugs		
temazepam	20 mg nocte	10–60 mg nocte
triazolam	0.25 mg	0.125–0.5 mg
diazepam	10 mg nocte	2 mg nocte–20 mg q4h
haloperidol	1.5 mg nocte	1.5–30 mg a day
chlorpromazine	25 mg q8h	10 mg nocte–150 mg q8h
amitriptyline	50 mg nocte	25 mg–150 mg nocte
clomipramine ⎱ dothiepin* ⎰	75 mg nocte	50–150 mg nocte
Anticonvulsants		
phenytoin	200 mg nocte	100–300 mg nocte
carbamazepine	200 mg b.i.d.	200 mg b.i.d.–400 mg t.i.d.
sodium valproate	500 mg nocte	200–1500 mg nocte

[1] Starting dose is often lower than modal dose: it is necessary to optimize dose before rejecting as ineffectual.
[2] Excluding 'as required' use.

INDEX

Note: Trade names are entered in *italics*, followed by the generic or product name.

Anticonvulsants, 99, 113, 114, 115,
178, 222
for deafferentation pain, 18, 34,
35, 36
Antidepressives, 48, 84, 101,
116–121, 178, 179, 185
anticholinergic effects of,
102–103
pain threshold and, 14
Antidiuretic hormone, 89–91
Antiemetics, 48, 60–61, 67, 68, 221
with opioids, 21, 24, 186–188, 196
see also individual drugs
Antiflatulents, 62, 63, 65, 133, 177,
194
Antihistamines, 60, 61, 125, 194
effects of, 43, 66, 70, 102–103,
143
pruritus and, 4, 148, 150, 194
see also individual drugs
Antihypertensives, 84
AntiParkinsonians, 43, 95, 104,
105, 106, 109
Antipsychotics, 107, 108, 109–110
Antisialogogues, 53
Antispasmodics, 43, 67, 102–103,
135, 136, 177
Antitussives, 126, 127
Anxiolytics, 101, 107, 108, 109,
110–113, 135
for dyspnoea, 131, 205
for pain relief, 14, 183, 185
for wakeful nights, 82, 179
APD (aminohydroxypropylidene
diphosphonate), 89, see
Pamidronate
Aphthous ulcer, 45
Arsenic, 99
Arthralgia, metastatic, 32
Arthritis, rheumatoid, 18
Arthropan (choline salicylate), 60
Ascites, 56, 78–79, 130, 131
Aserbine (desloughing agent), 159
Asilone (antiflatulent), 62, 63, 65,
133, 134
Aspirin, 19, 20, 22–23, 34, 151,
221
opioids with, 23, 177, 182
unwanted effects of, 22, 23, 59,
60
Asthma, 124, 130

Atarax (hydroxyzine), 150
Atelectasis, 130, 205
Atherosclerosis, cerebral, 97
Ativan (lorazepam), 112
Atropine, 136, 145
Auto-immune disease, 43
Aveeno Collodial (bath emollient),
152
Azo-Gantanol (phenazopyridine),
145
Azo-Gantrisin (phenazopyridine),
145

B & O Supprettes (belladonna and
opium), 136, 142
Baclofen, 106, 111
Bandaging, compression, 165, 168
Bandor adsorbent dressings, 159,
160
Barbiturates, 64, 83, 90, 99, 101
Barium, 75
Barrier cream, 153
Belladonna alkaloids, 43, 53, 66,
99, 136, 142
anticholinergic effects of,
102–103
Benorylate, 23, 221
Benzamides, 101
Benzocaine, 45, 142
Benzodiazepines, 101, 102,
110–115, 222
hyoscine and, 136
infusion of, 26, 97
paradoxical response to, 102,
107, 113
unwanted effects of, 56, 99, 111,
189
uses for, 33, 82, 110–111, 113,
114, 115, 179, 183
in akathisia, 104
as anticonvulsant, 113, 114, 115
as antiemetic, 60, 61, 113
in confusion, 96–97
in dementia, 106
in faecal impaction, 76
in respiratory symptoms, 131,
132, 205
in tardive dyskinesia, 106
Benzoin tincture, 125
Benzonatate, 126, 127, 134
Benzoyl peroxide, 160–161

Pupil dilation, 94
Pylorus, 68
Pyrexia, 128, 131, 191
Pyridium (phenazopyridine), 141,
143, 145
Pyridostigmine, 144

Questran (cholestyramine), 151
Quick Kwell (hyoscine), 136, 142

Radiation therapy, 16, 17, 31–32,
219
bone pain and, 18, 31, 32, 177,
203
drug doses following, 21, 32
dysphagia and, 53
fibrosis, 52, 65, 124, 130, 141
incontinence, 139
lymphoedema, 163, 164
nausea, 59, 61
oral, 42, 43, 46
unwanted effects of, 48, 50, 76, 84
Ranitidine, 57, 64
Rash, drug-induced, 150
Rectum
discharge from, 32, 75, 76–77
faeces impacted in, 58, 65, 71,
74–76, 138, 191
tenesmoid pain of, 107, 108, 135
ulceration of, 32
Reflux, 54, 56–57, 61, 62
Regulan (ispaghula), 72
Relatives, *see* Family
Religion, 209, 213
Renal, *see* Kidney
Reserpine, 106, 107
Respiratory symptoms, 3, 78,
123–135, 136, 175, 210
see also Bronchus
Restlessness, 94, 117, 121, 155
Restoril (temazepam), 82, 111
Retching, 58
Retroperitoneum, 65
Rheumatoid arthritis, 18
Ricinoleic acid, 72
Ripple air bed, 155
Robitussin (guaiphenesin), 125
Roho air bed, 155
Roxanol (morphine sulphate), 21,
22, 176

Rubber, skin allergy to, 148

Salicylates, non-acetylated, 23,
221
Saliva Substitute (artificial saliva),
42, 44
Salsalate, 23
Saran Wrap plastic film, 161
Sarcoid, 43
Sarcoidosis, 87, 99
Sarcoma, 91
Scabies, 148, 149
Scopaderm (hyoscine), 136
Scopolamine, *see* Hyoscine
Sears camping mattress, 155, 156
Second Skin (semipermeable
membrane), 158
Sedatives, 82–83, 84
benzodiazepines, 82, 110, 111,
113, 114, 115
haloperidol, 109
hyoscine, 135
morphine, 175, 179, 206
phenothiazines, 107, 108, 109
tricyclic drugs, 82, 117, 118, 119,
120
unwanted effects of, 95, 96, 140
Semipermeable membranes, 158
Senna, 24, 71, 72, 191, 222
Sennoside, 73, 74
Senokot (sennoside), 73, 74
Septicaemia, 189
Serenid (oxazepam), 112
Serotonin, 117, 118, 119, 120
Sialorrhoea, 53, 103, 135
Simethicone, *see* Dimethicone,
activated
Skin care, 147–161
in cachexia, 51
in lymphoedema, 165, 166–168
in pruritus, 4, 149–151
in rectal discharge, 77–78
see also Dry skin; Wet skin
Sodium bicarbonate, 62, 63
Sodium hypochlorite, 46, 159
Sodium phosphate, 72
Sodium sulphate, 72
Sodium valproate, 34, 35, 106, 134
doses of, 222
Soft tissue pain, 12, 18, 19
Solvents, organic, 99